I0788923

Culinary dictionary for lose weight

Cédric MENARD
DIETICIAN-NUTRITIONIST

Note: this book is strictly and only adapted for lose weight. This book is not adapted to any intolerance or food allergy.

ISBN: 9798698671022

Traduced by Mélanie GEFFROY

Legend of this book

- The searched word is **edible <u>without any limitation</u>** because it has a neutral role. In this case, it will have **three full stars** ★ ★ ★.

- The searched word is **edible** in moderation. Indeed, it is more or less likely to trigger disorders, more or less directly or indirectly linked to your health problem. In this case, it will have **two full stars** ★ ★.

- The searched word is **edible, but in great moderation**. In this case, it will have **one full star** ★. In the best case scenario, do not eat it.

- The searched word is **greatly not recommended**, not to say forbidden. It will be designated by this type of grey frame.

A

Abalone★★★/*Ormeau*: edible saltwater mollusk.

Abondance cheese★/*Abondance*: semi-hard and raw cow's milk cheese.
Note: do not consume more than approximately ½ oz of cheese three times per week... and never at dinner.

Accra/*Acra*: croquette of crushed cod or other various elements coated with fritter batter and fried in boiling oil.

Achars★★★/*Achards*: Indian condiment made of fruits and vegetables macerated in vinegar.

Adzuki bean/*Haricot azukis*: cf. "Kidney bean".

Adzuki flake★★★/*Flocon d'azukis*: small portion of dehydrated adzuki. Gluten-free.

Agar-agar★★★/*Agar-agar*: mucilage made from seaweed used as setting agent.

Agave syrup★/*Sirop d'agave*: syrup considered as a sweetener made of agave.

Aiguillette★★/*Aiguillette*: beef meat to roast. Red meat.
Note: do not consume more than approximately 4 oz of red meat twice per week. Cook it without fat: en papillote, in water, grill, roast...

Aillade★★★/*Aillade*: bread crouton rubbed with garlic and moistened with olive oil. Carbohydrate.

Alcohol (alcoholic beverage)★/*Alcool (boisson alcoolisée)*: wine, liqueur, beer, etc. made from alcohol fermentation.
Note: do not drink alcoholic beverage, however no problem if it's cooked.

Alcohol-free beer/*Bière sans alcool*: drink from the alcoholic fermentation of mainly barley and from which the alcohol is extracted.

Alexanders★★★/*Maceron*: plant from which we eat the young blanched shoots. Green vegetable.

Alfalfa seed★★★/*Graine d'alfalfa*: alfalfa seeds eaten crushed or germinated.

Alliaria★★★/*Alliaire*: plant with white flowers, garlic scent and spicy taste.

Almond★★/*Amande*: seed of the almond tree.

Almond butter★/*Beurre d'amande*: food paste made of grilled almonds.

Almond cream★★★/*Crème d'amande*: more or less liquid cream made of almond milk, substitute to crème fraîche.

Almond milk★★★/*Lait d'amande*: plant milk from almonds. Lactose-free.
Note: do not consume if it's sweetened.

Almond milk cream dessert/*Crème dessert au lait d'amande*: vegetable dessert made of almond milk, sugar and eggs. Dairy product.

Almond milk yogurt★★★/*Yaourt au lait d'amande*: almond milk fermented thanks to lactic acid bacteria, sweetened or not. Dairy product. Lactose-free.
Note: do not consume if it's sweetened.

Almond oil★★/***Huile d'amande***: fatty substance made of almond.

Almond pasta★★★/***Pâte alimentaire à base d'amande***: mix to be cooked made of sieved almond flour. Gluten-free.

Almond purée★★/***Purée d'amande***: mashed almonds to spread.
Note: do not consume if it's sweetened.

Almond seed★★/***Graine d'amande***: almond seed eaten crushed or germinated.

Almond syrup★★★/***Orgeat***: almond milk with orange blossom.
Note: do not consume if it's sweetened.

Amandine/*Amandine*: almond tartlet.

Amaranth★★★/***Amarante***: vegetable plant from which we eat the young leaves. Green vegetable.

Amaranth flour★★★/***Farine d'amarante***: powder made of not wholewheat amaranth milling. Gluten-free.

Amaranth pasta★★★/***Pâte alimentaire à base d'amarante***: mix to be cooked made of not whole-grain amaranth flour. Gluten-free.

Amaranth seed★★★/***Graine d'amarante***: amaranth seed eaten crushed or germinated.

American cheese★: melted cheese. Dairy product.
Note: do not consume more than approximately ½ oz of cheese three times per week... and never at dinner.

Anchoïade★★/***Anchoïade***: anchovy and olive oil purée.

Anchovy★★★/***Anchois***: small fatty saltwater fish.

Anchovy cream - Apple in light syrup

Anchovy cream★★/*Crème d'anchois*: mixed anchovies with olive oil.

Anchovy in oil★★/*Anchois à l'huile*: anchovy fillet preserved in vegetable oil.

Andouille/*Andouille*: product made of cooked cold meat, wrapped in black entrails, especially made from pork.

Andouillette★/*Andouillette*: cooked cold meat wrapped in entrails, especially made from pork.
Note: cook it without fat: to grill, to roast, etc.

Angelica★★★/*Angélique*: aromatic umbellifer plant.

Angler fish★★★/*Lotte*: saltwater or freshwater fish with white flesh.
Note: cook it without fat: en papillote, in water, grill...

Angler fish liver★★★/*Foie de lotte*: liver of the angler fish, saltwater fish. Offal.

Anise★★★/*Anis*: fruit used to flavor some alcoholic beverages, dishes, etc.

Appelwood cheese★: raw or pasteurised cow's milk cheese. Dairy product.
Note: do not consume more than approximately ½ oz of cheese three times per week... and never at dinner.

Appenzeller cheese★/*Appenzel*: hard cow's milk Swiss cheese. Dairy product.
Note: do not consume more than approximately ½ oz of cheese three times per week... and never at dinner.

Appetizer/*Amuse-gueule*: small salty cake, canapé, etc.

Apple in light syrup/*Pomme au sirop léger*: poached apple preserved in more or less sugary water.

Apple in syrup/*Pomme au sirop*: poached apple preserved in very sugary water.

Apple juice★/*Jus de pomme*: juice made of the pressing of apples.

Apricot in light syrup/*Abricot au sirop léger*: poached apricot preserved in more or less sugary water.

Apricot in syrup/*Abricot au sirop*: poached apricot preserved in very sugary water.

Apricot jelly/*Pâte d'abricot*: cf. "Dried apricot".

Apricot juice★/*Jus d'abricot*: juice made of the pressing of apricots.

Arctic char★★★/*Omble*: fatty freshwater fish.
Note: cook it without fat: en papillote, in water, grill...

Arctostaphylos uva-ursi★★★/*Busserole*: small edible berry from a bush: the arctostaphylos uva-ursi tree. Fresh fruit.

Argan oil★★/*Huile d'argan*: fatty substance made of argan.

Aronia in might syrup/*Aronia au sirop léger*: poached aronia preserved in more or less sugary water.

Aronia in syrup/*Aronia au sirop*: poached aronia preserved in very sugary water.

Artichoke★★★/*Artichaut*: vegetable perennial plant grown for its flower heads from which we eat the bract. Green vegetable.

Arugula★★★/*Roquette*: annual plant from which the prickly leaves are eaten in salad. Green vegetable.

Arugula seed - Ayrshire cheese

Arugula seed★★★/*Graine de roquette*: arugula seed eaten crushed or germinated.

Asiago★/*Asiago*: Italian hard cow's milk cheese. Dairy product.
Note: do not consume more than approximately ½ oz of cheese three times per week... and never at dinner.

Asparagus★★★/*Asperge*: vegetable plant grown for its young shoots. Green vegetables.

Asparagus pea★★★/*Pois-asperge*: vegetable plant from which we eat the cloves and the seeds. Green vegetable.

Aspartame★★★/*Aspartame*: intense artificial sweetener with no calorie.

Aspic★★★/*Aspic*: dish coated with jelly.

Asses' milk/*Lait d'ânesse*: whole milk from the she-ass.

Atlantic horse mackerel★★★/*Chinchard*: fatty saltwater fish.
Note: cook it without fat: en papillote, in water, grill, roast...

Atriplex hortensis★★★/*Arroche*: plant with triangular leaves. Only one species is edible. Green vegetable.

Avocado★/*Avocat*: oleaginous fruit of the avocado tree.

Avocado oil★★/*Huile d'avocat*: fatty substance made of avocado.

Ayrshire cheese★: raw or pasteurised cow's milk cheese. Dairy product.
Note: do not consume more than approximately ½ oz of cheese three times per week... and never at dinner.

Azerole in light syrup/*Azerole au sirop léger*: poached azerole preserved in more or less sugary water.

Azerole in powder★★★/*Azerole en poudre*: azerole extracts sold in capsules or in tablets.

Azerole in syrup/*Azerole au sirop*: poached azerole preserved in sugary water.

B

Babelutte/*Babelutte*: candy cane flavored with honey or brown sugar.

Baby-beef★★/*Baby-beef*: young bovine fattened for its meat, slaughtered between 12 and 15 months. Red meat.
Note: do not consume more than approximately 4 oz of red meat twice per week. Cook it without fat: en papillote, in water, grill, roast...

Bacon★★★/*Bacon*: piece of pork carcass salted and smoked, cut in thin slices. Cooked meat.

Bagel★★/*Bagel*: small white bread shaped into a ring with very firm crumb. Carbohydrate.

Bagnes cheese★/*Bagnes*: hard unpasteurized cow's milk cheese. Dairy product.
Note: do not consume more than approximately ½ oz of cheese three times per week... and never at dinner.

Baguette/*Baguette*: white bread that has a high glycemic index. Carbohydrate.

Baker's yeast★★★/*Levure de boulanger*: unicellular microscopic mushrooms used for the bread batter fermentation.

Baking powder★★★/*Levure chimique*: mix of chemical products used in pastry cooking and in cookie cooking to make the batter rise.

Baking soda★★★/*Bicarbonate de soude*: cf. "Bicarbonate of soda".

Baklava/*Baklava*: small Turkish cake with puff pastry, honey and almonds.

Ballan wrasse★★★/*Vieille*: saltwater fish with white flesh.
Note: cook it without fat: en papillote, in water, grill, roast...

Ballotine★/*Ballottine*: rolled galantine with poultry and stuffing. Cooked meat.

Bambara nut★★★/*Pois de bambara*: ground-bean. Carbohydrate. Gluten-free.

Bamboo (shoot of)★★★/*Bambou (pousses de)*: young shoots of edible bamboo. Green vegetable.

Banana juice/*Jus de banane*: juice made of the pressing of bananas. Exotic fruit.

Banana split/*Banana split*: dessert made of banana, vanilla ice cream, whipped cream and almonds. Exotic fruit.

Banana★★★/*Banane tigrée*: tropical fruit of the banana tree, rich in starch before its full ripeness. Exotic fruit.
Note: do not consume ripe banana.

Banon cheese★/*Banon*: unpasteurized goat or sheep milk wrapped in a sweet chestnut leaf. Dairy product.
Note: do not consume more than approximately ½ oz of cheese three times per week... and never at dinner.

Barb★★★/*Barbeau*: freshwater fish with white flesh.
Note: cook it without fat: en papillote, in water, grill, roast...

Barbecue sauce/*Sauce barbecue*: sauce mainly made of sugar, flavors and tomato purée.

Bard/*Barde*: lard slice used to wrap a piece of poultry or a piece of meat.

Barley flake★★★/*Flocon d'orge*: small portion of dehydrated barley. Carbohydrate.

Barley milk★★★/*Lait d'orge*: plant milk from barley. Lactose-free.
Note: do not consume if it's sweetened.

Barley milk cream dessert/*Crème dessert au lait d'orge*: vegetable dessert made of barley milk, sugar and eggs. Dairy product.

Barley pasta★★★/*Pâte alimentaire d'orge*: mix to be cooked made of refined barley flour. Carbohydrate.

Barracuda★★★/*Barracuda*: saltwater fish with white flesh.
Note: cook it without fat: en papillote, in water, grill, roast...

Basil★★★/*Basilic*: herb you can use as a condiment.

Basil seed★★★/*Graine de basilic*: basil seed eaten crushed or germinated.

Basquaise sauce★★★/*Sauce basquaise*: sauce made of tomatoes, onions, bell peppers, olives and Espelette chili peppers.

Bass★★★/*Bar*: saltwater fish with white flesh.
Note: cook it without fat: en papillote, in water, grill, roast...

Batavia lettuce - Beef fondue

Batavia lettuce★★★/*Batavia*: lettuce with crunchy leaves. Green vegetable.

Bavarian cream/*Bavarois*: dessert with custard and gelatin.

Bay★★★/*Laurier-sauce*: aromatic leaf used as a condiment.

Bearnaise sauce/*Sauce béarnaise*: sauce made of egg yolks, garlics, shallots, tarragons and butter.

Beaufort cheese★/*Beaufort*: firm raw cow's milk cheese. Dairy product.
Note: do not consume more than approximately ½ oz of cheese three times per week... and never at dinner.

Béchamel sauce★★★/*Sauce béchamel*: white sauce made of a roux and milk.

Beef breast★/*Poitrine de bœuf*: inferior part of the beef's rib cage to boil. Red meat.
Note: do not consume more than approximately 4 oz of red meat twice per week. Cook it without fat.

Beef carpaccio★★/*Carpaccio de bœuf*: beef meat cut in very thin slices eaten raw, with a drop of olive oil and lemon juice. Red meat.
Note: do not consume more than approximately 4 oz of red meat twice per week.

Beef cheek★★/*Joue de bœuf*: tender piece of beef cooked in sauce. Red meat.
Note: do not consume more than approximately 4 oz of red meat twice per week. Cook it without fat.

Beef fondue/*Fondue bourguignonne*: dish made of small dices of beef dipped in boiling oil. Red meat.

Beef gristle★★/*Tendron de bœuf*: part of the beef composed of the cartilages which prolong the ribs. Red meat.
Note: do not consume more than approximately 4 oz of red meat twice per week. Cook it without fat: en papillote, in water, grill, roast...

Beef kidney★★/*Rognon de bœuf*: kidney of the beef. Offal.
Note: cook it without fat: to grill, to roast, etc.

Beef knuckle★★/*Jarret de bœuf*: part of the leg behind the beef's knee joint. Meat to boil. Red meat.
Note: do not consume more than approximately 4 oz of red meat twice per week. Cook it without fat.

Beef liver★★/*Foie de bœuf*: offal.
Note: cook it without fat: to grill, to roast, etc.

Beef (meat)★★/*Bœuf (viande de)*: all unprepared nor transformed meats, plain, ready to be cooked and cut from beef.
Note: do not consume more than approximately 4 oz of red meat twice per week. Cook it without fat: en papillote, in water, grill, roast...

Beef ravioli★★★/*Ravioli de bœuf*: small square of pasta stuffed with beef meat, ground herbs, etc. before being poached. Carbohydrate.

Beef short ribs★/*Plat de côte (de bœuf)*: beef meat to boil.

Beef spare rib★★/*Echine de bœuf*: part of the beef consisting of the ribs and the sirloin. Red meat.
Note: do not consume more than approximately 4 oz of red meat twice per week. Cook it without fat: en papillote, in water, grill, roast...

Beef spider steak★★/*Araignée de bœuf*: piece of very tender meat from the beef's pelvis muscles. Red meat.
Note: do not consume more than approximately 4 oz of red meat twice per week. Cook it without fat: en papillote, in water, grill, roast...

Beef steak★★/*Bifteck*: slice of beef to grill. Red meat.
Note: do not consume more than approximately 4 oz of red meat twice per week.

Beef stock★★★/*Fond de bœuf*: brown stock made of beef stock.

Beef surlonge★★/*Surlonge de bœuf*: piece of beef to simmer. Red meat.
Note: do not consume more than approximately 4 oz of red meat twice per week. Cook it without fat.

Beef tongue★★★/*Langue de bœuf*: beef tongue eaten boiled. Offal.

Beef tournedos★★/*Tournedos de bœuf*: round slice of beef fillet. Red meat.
Note: do not consume more than approximately 4 oz of red meat twice per week. Cook it without fat: en papillote, in water, grill, roast...

Beer★/*Bière*: beverage from alcoholic fermentation, especially barley alcoholic fermentation.
Note: do not drink alcoholic beverage, however no problem if it's cooked.

Beet★★★/*Betterave*: vegetable plant from which we eat the plump root. Green vegetable.

Beetroot chips/*Chips de betterave*: very thinly cut beetroots, fried and salted.

Beet seed★★★/*Graine de betterave*: beet seed eaten crushed or germinated.

Bell pepper★★★/*Poivron*: soft bell pepper. Green vegetable.

Bicarbonate of soda★★★/*Bicarbonate de sodium*: basic sodium salt sometimes used to ease stomach aches.

Bison (meat)★★/*Bison (viande de)*: meat very similar to that of beef. Red meat.
Note: do not consume more than approximately 4 oz of red meat twice per week. Cook it without fat: en papillote, in water, grill, roast...

Bisque★★★/*Bisque*: soup made of crustacean coulis.

Black ascophyllum★★★/*Goémon noir*: edible seaweed.

Blackberry in light syrup/*Mûre au sirop léger*: poached blackberry preserved in more or less sugary water.

Blackberry in syrup/*Mûre au sirop*: poached blackberry preserved in very sugary water.

Black bread★★★/*Pain noir*: bread made of wheat flour, buckwheat flour, rye flour. Carbohydrate.

Blackcurrant in light syrup/*Cassis au sirop léger*: poached blackcurrant preserved in more or less sugary water.

Blackcurrant in syrup/*Cassis au sirop*: poached blackcurrant preserved in very sugary water.

Black radish seed★★★/*Graine de radis noir*: black radish seed eaten crushed or germinated.

Black sausage/*Boudin noir*: cooked cold meat made of pork blood and fat stuffed in an intestine.

Black tea★★★/***Thé noir***: infusion of tea bush leaves lightly fermented after being picked.
Note: do not drink it sweetened.

Black turtle bean★★★/***Haricot noir***: black bean seed eaten fully ripe. Carbohydrate.

Blanquette★/***Blanquette***: dish made of boiled meat (veal, turkey, lamb) served with a sauce made of stock thickened with flour and butter.

Bleak★★★/***Ablette***: small freshwater fish with white flesh.
Note: cook it without fat: en papillote, in water, to grill. Do not fry.

Blended yogurt/***Yaourt brassé***: cf. "Yogurt".

Blengdale blue★: raw or pasteurised cow's milk cheese. Dairy product.
Note: do not consume more than approximately ½ oz of cheese three times per week... and never at dinner.

Bleu de Gex★/***Septmoncel***: cow's milk cheese with mildew in it.
Note: do not consume more than approximately ½ oz of cheese three times per week... and never at dinner.

Bleu du Vercors-Sassenage★/***Sassenage***: hard cow's milk cheese with internal mildew. Dairy product.
Note: do not consume more than approximately ½ oz of cheese three times per week... and never at dinner.

Bliblis★★★/***Bliblis***: grilled chickpeas. Carbohydrate. Gluten-free.

Blinis★★★/***Blini***: small wheat and buckwheat crepe. Carbohydrate.
Note: do not consume if it's sweetened.

Blitum bonus-henricus★★★/*Ansérine bon-henri*: vegetable plant from which we eat the young leaves. Green vegetable.

Blonchester cheese★: raw or pasteurised cow's milk cheese. Dairy product.
Note: do not consume more than approximately ½ oz of cheese three times per week... and never at dinner.

Blood orange/*Orange sanguine*: cf. "Orange".

Blood orange juice★/*Jus d'orange sanguine*: juice made of the pressing of blood oranges.

Bloody Mary/*Bloody Mary*: cocktail with vodka and tomato juice.

Blueberry in light syrup/*Myrtille au sirop léger*: poached blueberry preserved in more or less sugary water.

Blueberry in syrup/*Myrtille au sirop*: poached blueberry preserved in very sugary water.

Blueberry juice★/*Jus de myrtille*: juice made of the pressing of blueberries.

Blue cheese★/*Bleu*: blue-veined aged cheese. Dairy product. Blue marble Jack, Maytag blue...
Note: do not consume more than approximately ½ oz of cheese three times per week... and never at dinner.

Blue marble Jack★: pasteurised cow's milk cheese. Dairy product.
Note: do not consume more than approximately ½ oz of cheese three times per week... and never at dinner.

Boeuf bourguignon★★/*Bourguignon (bœuf)*: beef stew with red wine and onions. Red meat.
Note: do not consume more than approximately 4 oz of red meat twice per week. Cook it without fat, or only with olive oil

Bogue★★★/*Bogue*: saltwater fish with white flesh.
Note: cook it without fat: en papillote, in water, grill, roast...

Bolognese sauce★★/*Sauce bolognaise*: sauce made of tomatoes, onions and ground meat (usually beef meat, so red meat).

Borage★★★/*Bourrache officinale*: plant you can use as condiment and from which we eat the young leaves.

Bouillabaisse★★★/*Bouillabaisse*: soup made of various fish, crustacea, etc.

Brains★★/*Cervelle*: brain of some animals intended to be eaten.

Braised (cooking method)★★/*Braisé (cuisson en)*: cooking method consisting in cooking food in a very flavored and low-fat or even no fat at all base, in isolation.

Braised ham★★★/*Jambon braisé*: pork ham juged in a braising base.
Note: cook it without fat: to grill, to roast, etc.

Bran bread/*Pain de son*: cf. "Wholewheat bread".

Brandade★★★/*Brandade*: dish made of cod and potatoes.

Brazil nut/*Noix du Brésil*: cf. "Nut".

Bread★★★/*Paner*: to coat a food with a mixture of whipped egg and breadcrumbs before cooking it.

Breadcrumbs★★★/*Chapelure*: white bread toasted in the oven before being crushed into crumbs. Carbohydrate.

Breaded breast of lamb★★/*Epigramme d'agneau*: high part of the cutlet. Red meat.
Note: do not consume more than approximately 4 oz of red meat twice per week. Cook it without fat: en papillote, in water, grill, roast...

Breaded fish★★★/*Poisson pané*: fish with white flesh coated with breadcrumbs.
Note: cook it without fat.

Breaded knuckle of ham★★★/*Jambonneau pané*: part of the leg above the knee breaded with wheat breadcrumbs. Cooked meat.

Breaded meat★★★/*Viande panée*: meat coated with breadcrumbs.
Note: breaded red meat are★★. Do not cook with fat.

Breadfruit★★/*Fruit à pain*: fruit from the breadfruit tree.

Bread with dried fruits★★/*Pain aux fruits secs*: bread enriched with dried fruits. Carbohydrate.

Bread with grains★★★/*Pain aux graines*: wholewheat bread with crushed or whole grains. Carbohydrate.

Breakfast cookie/*Biscuit pour petit-déjeuner*: cookie adapted to breakfast, rich in cereals. Carbohydrate.

Breakfast sugary extruded cereal/*Céréale extrudée sucrée pour petit-déjeuner*: swelled cereal coated in sugar, honey, chocolat, etc. Carbohydrate.

Bream★★★/*Brème*: freshwater fish with white flesh.
Note: cook it without fat: en papillote, in water, grill, roast...

Breckland thyme★★★/*Serpolet*: plant used as a condiment.

Brewer's yeast★★★/*Levure de bière*: unicellular microscopic mushrooms.

Brick cheese★: pasteurised cow's milk cheese. Dairy product.
Note: do not consume more than approximately ½ oz of cheese three times per week... and never at dinner.

Brie cheese★/*Brie*: soft aged cow's milk cheese with bloomy rind. Dairy product.
Note: do not consume more than approximately ½ oz of cheese three times per week... and never at dinner.

Brill★★★/*Barbue*: saltwater fish with white flesh.
Note: cook it without fat: en papillote, in water, grill, roast...

Brillat-savarin cheese★/*Brillat-savarin*: soft raw cow's milk cheese with bloomy rind. Triple cream cheese. Dairy product.
Note: do not consume more than approximately ½ oz of cheese three times per week... and never at dinner.

Brined anchovy★★★/*Anchois en saumure*: anchovy fillet preserved in salt.

Brioche/*Brioche*: puffy pastry made of flour, yeast, fats and eggs.

Brioche bread/*Pain brioché*: cf. "Brioche".

Brioche crispbread/*Biscotte briochée*: slice of brioche sandwich bread industrially toasted in the oven. Carbohydrate.

Brocciu★/*Broccio*: goat or sheep milk cheese. Dairy product.
Note: do not consume more than approximately ½ oz of cheese three times per week... and never at dinner.

Broccoli★★★/*Chou brocoli*: cabbage from which we eat the central inflorescence.

Broccoli seed★★★/*Graine de chou brocoli*: broccoli seed eaten crushed or germinated.

Broth★★★/*Bouillon*: light soup made by boiling meat and vegetables in water.

Brouillade★★★/*Brouillade*: dish made of scrambled eggs.

Brousse★★★/*Brousse*: whey cheese made of goat, sheep or cow's milk very similar to ricotta. Dairy product.

Brown butter/*Beurre noisette*: butter heated until brown in a pan.

Brownie/*Brownie*: small chocolate cake with walnuts.

Brown mustard with cabbage leaf★★★/*Moutarde de Chine à feuille de chou*: vegetable plant from which we eat the leaves. Green vegetable.

Brown rice pasta/*Pâte alimentaire de riz brun*: cf. "Whole-grain rice pasta".

Brown sugar/*Sucre roux*: cane sugar which kept its impurities.

Brussel sprouts★★★/*Chou de Bruxelles*: vegetable plant from which we only eat the flower heads on the main stem.

Buckling★★★/*Hareng saur*: salted herring smoked thanks to smoke.
Note: cook it without fat: en papillote, grill, roast...

Buckwheat bulgur★★★/*Boulgour de sarrasin*: sieved and crushed buckwheat steamed or cooked in water. Carbohydrate. Gluten-free.

Buckwheat cornflakes★★★**/Corn flakes de sarrasin**: grilled flakes made of sieved buckwheat flakes. Carbohydrate. Gluten-free.
Note: do not consume if it's sweetened.

Buckwheat cream★★★**/Crème de sarrasin**: more or less liquid cream made of buckwheat milk, substitute to crème fraîche.

Buckwheat flake★★★**/Flocon de sarrasin**: small portion of dehydrated buckwheat. Carbohydrate.
Note: do not consume if it's sweetened.

Buckwheat milk★★★**/Lait de sarrasin**: plant milk from buckwheat. Lactose-free.
Note: do not consume if it's sweetened.

Buckwheat milk cream dessert/Crème dessert au lait de sarrasin: vegetable dessert made of buckwheat milk, sugar and eggs.

Buckwheat pancake★★★**/Galette**: flat, thin and round dish made of buckwheat flour, eggs and milk cooked in a frying pan. Carbohydrate. Gluten-free.

Buckwheat pasta★★★**/Pâte alimentaire de sarrasin**: mix to be cooked made of refined buckwheat flour. Carbohydrate.

Buffalo/Buffle: cf. "Beef (meat)".

Bulgur★★★**/Boulgour**: sieved and crushed wheat steamed or cooked in water. Carbohydrate.

Bun★★**/Bun**: small round and puffy white bread. Carbohydrate.

Burger★**/Burger**: round sandwich used as a staple in fast food restaurants. Carbohydrate.

Burger sauce/*Sauce burger*: sauce mainly made of vegetable oil, flavors, sugar and tomato purée.

Buttermilk★★★/*Babeurre*: liquid residue obtained after churning butter out of cream.

Button mangosteen in light syrup/*Mangoustan au sirop léger*: poached button mangosteen preserved in more or less sugary water. Exotic fruit.

Button mangosteen in syrup/*Mangoustan au sirop*: poached button mangosteen preserved in very sugary water. Exotic fruit.

Button mangosteen juice/*Jus de mangoustan*: juice made of the pressing of button mangosteens. Exotic fruit.

Button mushroom★★★/*Champignon de Paris*: small edible white mushroom.

Buxton blue★: raw or pasteurised cow's milk cheese. Dairy product.
Note: do not consume more than approximately ½ oz of cheese three times per week... and never at dinner.

C

Cabbage (red, white, green)★★★/*Chou pommé (rouge, blanc, vert)*: vegetable plant from which we eat the leaves.

Cachou/*Cachou*: aromatic pastille flavored with areca nut.

Caerphilly cheese★: raw or pasteurised cow's milk cheese. Dairy product.
Note: do not consume more than approximately ½ oz of cheese three times per week... and never at dinner.

Café liégeois - Candied banana

Café liégeois/*Liégeois (café)*: coffee ice cream coated with whipped cream.

Cake/*Gâteau*: pastry made of a batter used alone or with a cream, fruits, sugar...

Calf's head/*Tête de veau*: calf's head eaten boiled. Offal.

Calisson/*Calisson*: candy in a diamond shape made of almonds and which top is frosted.

Camelina sativa oil★★/*Huile de cameline*: fatty substance made of camelina sativa.

Camembert★/*Camembert*: aged soft cow's milk cheese with bloomy rind. Dairy product.
Note: do not consume more than approximately ½ oz of cheese three times per week... and never at dinner.

Canapé★/*Canapé*: small slice of sandwich bread on which various mixtures are spread. Carbohydrate.
Note: do not consume if it's sweetened and/or too fat.

Cancoillotte★★★/*Cancoillotte*: low-fat melted cow's milk cheese. Dairy product.

Candied apple/*Pomme confite*: apple preserved thanks to the replacement of its water by sugar.

Candied apricot/*Abricot confit*: fresh apricot greatly enriched with sugar.

Candied aronia/*Aronia confite*: aronia preserved thanks to the replacement of its water by sugar.

Candied azerole/*Azerole confite*: azerole preserved thanks to the replacement of its water by sugar.

Candied banana/*Banane confite*: banana preserved thanks to the replacement of its water by sugar. Exotic fruit.

Candied blackberry/*Mûre confite*:   blackberry preserved thanks to the replacement of its water by sugar.

Candied blackcurrant/*Cassis confit*: blackcurrant berry preserved thanks to the replacement of its water by sugar.

Candied blueberry/*Myrtille confite*:   blueberry preserved thanks to the replacement of its water by sugar.

Candied button mangosteen/*Mangoustan confit*: button mangosteen preserved thanks to the replacement of its water by sugar. Exotic fruit.

Candied carambola/*Carambole confite*: carambola preserved thanks to the replacement of its water by sugar. Exotic fruit.

Candied cherimoya/*Anone confite*:   cherimoya preserved thanks to the replacement of its water by sugar. Exotic fruit.

Candied cherry/*Cerise confite*:   cherry preserved thanks to the replacement of its water by sugar.

Candied chestnut/*Marron glacé*: chestnut candied in sugar and iced with syrup.

Candied chili pepper in vinegar★★★/*Piment confit au vinaigre*: chili pepper preserved in vinegar. Green vegetable.

Candied clementine/*Clémentine confite*: clementine preserved thanks to the replacement of its water by sugar.

Candied coconut/*Noix de coco confite*: coconut pulp preserved thanks to the replacement of its water by sugar. Exotic fruit.

Candied cocoplum/*Icaque confit*: cocoplum preserved thanks to the replacement of its water by sugar. Exotic fruit.

Candied cranberry/*Canneberge confite*: cranberry preserved thanks to the replacement of its water by sugar.

Candied date/*Datte confite*: date preserved thanks to the replacement of its water by sugar. Exotic fruit.

Candied fig/*Figue confite*: fig preserved thanks to the replacement of its water by sugar.

Candied fruit/*Fruit confit*: fruit cooked in sugar syrup before being slowly dried.

Candied ginger/*Gingembre confit*: slice of ginger cooked and candied in sugar syrup.

Candied goji berry/*Baie de goji confite*: small red fruit eaten after being greatly enriched in sugar.

Candied grape/*Raisin confit*: grape preserved thanks to the replacement of its water by sugar.

Candied grapefruit/*Pamplemousse confit*: grapefruit preserved thanks to the replacement of its water by sugar.

Candied guava/*Goyave confite*: guava preserved thanks to the replacement of its water by sugar. Exotic fruit.

Candied jujube/*Jujube confite*: jujube preserved thanks to the replacement of its water by sugar. Exotic fruit.

Candied kaki/*Kaki confit*: kaki preserved thanks to the replacement of its water by sugar.

Candied kiwi/*Kiwi confit*: kiwi preserved thanks to the replacement of its water by sugar.

Candied kumquat/*Kumquat confit*: kumquat preserved thanks to the replacement of its water by sugar.

Candied lemon/*Citron confit*: lemon preserved thanks to the replacement of its water by sugar.

Candied longan/*Longane confite*: longan preserved thanks to the replacement of its water by sugar. Exotic fruit.

Candied lychee/*Litchi confit*: lychee preserved thanks to the replacement of its water by sugar. Exotic fruit.

Candied Malay rose apple/*Jambose confite*: Malay rose apple preserved thanks to the replacement of its water by sugar. Exotic fruit.

Candied mandarin/*Mandarine confite*: mandarin preserved thanks to the replacement of its water by sugar.

Candied mango/*Mangue confite*: mango preserved thanks to the replacement of its water by sugar. Exotic fruit.

Candied meat/*Viande confite*: cooked meat preserved in is fat.

Candied medlar/*Nèfle confite*: medlar preserved thanks to the replacement of its water by sugar.

Candied melon/*Melon confit*: melon preserved thanks to the replacement of its water by sugar.

Candied mirabelle plum/*Mirabelle confite*: mirabelle plum preserved thanks to the replacement of its water by sugar.

Candied mombins/*Mombin confit*: mombins preserved thanks to the replacement of its water by sugar. Exotic fruit.

Candied mulberries/*Mulberries confite*: mulberries preserved thanks to the replacement of its water by sugar.

Candied myrciaria/*Camu-camu confite*: myrciaria preserved thanks to the replacement of its water by sugar. Exotic fruit.

Candied orange/*Orange confite*: orange preserved thanks to the replacement of its water by sugar.

Candied papaya/*Papaye confite*: papaya preserved thanks to the replacement of its water by sugar. Exotic fruit.

Candied passion fruit/*Grenadille confite*: passion fruit preserved thanks to the replacement of its water by sugar. Exotic fruit.

Candied peach/*Pêche confite*: peach preserved thanks to the replacement of its water by sugar.

Candied pear/*Poire confite*: pear preserved thanks to the replacement of its water by sugar.

Candied physalis/*Physalis confite*: physalis preserved thanks to the replacement of its water by sugar. Exotic fruit.

Candied pineapple/*Ananas confit*: pineapple preserved thanks to the replacement of its water by sugar. Exotic fruit.

Candied plum/*Prune confite*: plum preserved thanks to the replacement of its water by sugar.

Candied quince/*Coing confit*: quince preserved thanks to the replacement of its water by sugar.

Candied rambutan/*Ramboutan confit*: rambutan preserved thanks to the replacement of its water by sugar. Exotic fruit.

Candied raspberry/*Framboise confite*: raspberry preserved thanks to the replacement of its water by sugar.

Candied redcurrant/*Groseille confite*: redcurrant preserved thanks to the replacement of its water by sugar.

Candied salak/*Salacca confit*: salak preserved thanks to the replacement of its water by sugar. Exotic fruit.

Candied sapodilla/*Sapotille confite*: sapodilla fruit preserved thanks to the replacement of its water by sugar. Exotic fruit.

Candied sloe/*Prunelle confite*: sloe preserved thanks to the replacement of its water by sugar.

Candied sorb/*Sorbe confite*: sorb preserved thanks to the replacement of its water by sugar.

Candied strawberry/*Fraise confite*: strawberry preserved thanks to the replacement of its water by sugar.

Candied tamarind fruit/*Tamarin confit*: tamarind fruit preserved thanks to the replacement of its water by sugar. Exotic fruit.

Candied vegetable★★★/*Légume confit*: green vegetable preserved in vinegar.

Candied watermelon/*Pastèque confite*: watermelon preserved thanks to the replacement of its water by sugar.

Candy/*Bonbon*: confection only made of sugar and flavor.

Candy cane/*Sucre d'orge*: stick of flavored and cooked sugar. Fast-acting sugar.

Cannellonis★★★/*Cannelloni*: wheat pasta rolled in the shape of a cylinder and stuffed with stuffing. Carbohydrate.

Canola oil★★/*Huile de colza*: fatty substance made of canola.

Cantal cheese★/*Cantal*: firm aged raw cow's milk cheese. Dairy product.
Note: do not consume more than approximately ½ oz of cheese three times per week... and never at dinner.

Cape gooseberry: cf. "Physalis peruviana".

Capelin - Caraway fruit

Capelin★★★/*Capelan*: saltwater fish with white flesh.
Note: cook it without fat: en papillote, in water, grill, roast...

Caper★★★/*Câpre*: condiment. Flower bud from the caper bush candied in vinegar.

Capocollo★/*Coppa*: cooked meat made of boned salted and smoked spare rib.

Capon★★★/*Chapon*: castrated cockerel. Poultry.
Note: cook it without fat: en papillote, in water, grill, roast...

Cappuccino★★★/*Cappuccino*: foaming coffee with milk.
Note: do not consume if it's sweetened.

Capricious cheese★: pasteurised goat's milk cheese. Dairy product.
Note: do not consume more than approximately ½ oz of cheese three times per week... and never at dinner.

Carambola in light syrup/*Carambole au sirop léger*: poached carambola preserved in more or less sugary water. Exotic fruit.

Carambola in syrup/*Carambole au sirop*: poached carambola preserved in very sugary water. Exotic fruit.

Caramel(1)/*Caramel(1)*: product made from the action of the heat on sugar mixed with a little bit of water.

Caramel(2)/*Caramel(2)*: candy made of sugar and fats (cream, milk, butter...)

Caraway fruit★★★/*Carvi*: aromatic fruit from the caraway (plain plant).

Carbohydrate/*Féculent*: food more or less rich in starch such as potatoes, dry beans (beans from Soissons, cranberry beans, navy beans, kidney beans, lentils, split peas, flageolets, etc.), pasta, rice, quinoa, bread, grains (wheat, barley, rye, oats, etc.) and their equivalents: bulgur, semolina, etc. flours (see various flours in the previous pages), starches (see above), cassava, sweet potatoes, fava beans, plantains, etc. (See each carbohydrate separately in this book).

Carbonara sauce/*Sauce carbonara*: sauce made of crème fraîche, parmesan cheese, egg yolks and aromatic herbs.

Cardoon★★★/*Cardon*: vegetable plant from which we eat the plump part of the leaves. Green vegetable.

Caribbean reef octopus★★★/*Chatrou*: small edible octopus.
Note: cook it without fat: en papillote, in water, grill, roast...

Carob powder★★★/*Poudre de caroube*: instant drink made of carob powder.
Note: do not consume if it's sweetened.

Carob seeds flour★★★/*Farine de graines de caroube*: powder made of carob seeds milling. Gluten-free.

Carp★★★/*Carpe*: freshwater fish with white flesh.
Note: cook it without fat: en papillote, in water, grill, roast...

Carré de l'Est★/*Carré de l'Est*: soft cow's milk cheese with bloomy rind. Dairy product.
Note: do not consume more than approximately ½ oz of cheese three times per week... and never at dinner.

Carrot★★★/*Carotte*: vegetable plant grown for its edible root. Green vegetable.

Carrot juice★★★/*Jus de carotte*: juice made of the pressing of carrots.

Carrots chips/*Chips de carottes*: very thinly cut carrots, fried and salted.

Carrot seed★★★/*Graine de carotte*: carrot seed eaten crushed or germinated.

Cashew milk★★★/*Lait de noix de cajou*: plant milk from cashews. Lactose-free.
Note: do not consume if it's sweetened.

Cashew nut★★/*Noix de cajou*: oleaginous seed from the cashew tree.

Cashew nut cream★★★/*Crème de noix de cajou*: more or less liquid cream made of cashew nut milk, substitute to crème fraîche.

Cashew nut milk cream dessert/*Crème dessert au lait de noix de cajou*: vegetable dessert made of cashew nut milk, sugar and eggs. Dairy product.

Cashew purée★★/*Purée de noix de cajou*: mashed cashews to spread.

Cassava/*Manioc*: cf. "Tapioca".

Cassava flake★★★/*Flocon de manioc*: small portion of dehydrated cassava. Carbohydrate. Gluten-free.

Cassava flour/*Farine de manioc*: cf. "Tapioca". Carbohydrate.

Cassava starch/*Fécule de manioc*: cf. "Tapioca". Carbohydrate.

Cassoulet★/*Cassoulet*: stew made of navy beans and goose confit, confit of duck, preserve of sheep or preserve of pork.

Castor oil★★/*Huile de ricin*: fatty substance made of castor seeds.

Catfish★★★/*Poisson-chat*: freshwater fish with white flesh.
Note: cook it without fat: en papillote, in water, grill, roast...

Cauliflower★★★/*Chou-fleur*: cabbage from which we eat the central inflorescence.

Caviar/*Caviar*: salt-cured roe.

Celeriac★★★/*Céleri-rave*: vegetable plant, kind of celery from which we eat the plump base. Green vegetable.

Celery★★★/*Céleri à couper*: vegetable plant from which we eat the petiole. Green vegetable.

Celery juice★★★/*Jus de céleri*: juice made of the pressing of celeries.

Celery salt★★★/*Sel de céleri*: celery in powder.

Celery seed★★★/*Graine de céleri*: celery seed eaten crushed or germinated.

Celery stick★★★/*Céleri branche*: vegetable plant from which we eat the petioles. Green vegetable.

Cereal bar/*Barre de céréales*: very sugary bar made of various cereals.

Cereal crispbread/*Biscotte aux céréales*: cf. "Wholegrain crispbread". Carbohydrate.

Cereals/*Céréales*: wheat, millet, oats, barley, rye, rice, corn, etc. For each cereal, see their own denomination. Carbohydrate.

Cervelas/*Cervelas*: cooked saucisson, cooked meat.

**Chabichou★/*Chabichou*: aged goat milk cheese. Dairy product.
Note: do not consume more than approximately ½ oz of cheese three times per week... and never at dinner.

**Chaerophyllum bulbosum★★★/*Cerfeuil tubéreux*: kind of chervil from which we eat the root. Green vegetable.

**Champagne/*Champagne*: sparkling white wine.

**Chaource cheese★★★/*Chaource*: soft cow's milk cheese with bloomy rind. Dairy product.

**Chard★★★/*Bette*: vegetable plant from which we eat the lines and leaves. Green vegetable.

**Chateaubriand★★/*Chateaubriand*: thick slice of grilled or stir fried beef fillet. Red meat.
Note: do not consume more than approximately 4 oz of red meat twice per week. Cook it without fat: grill, roast...

**Chayote★★/*Chayote*: fruit grown in warm countries and which has the same shape as a big green pear. Exotic fruit.

**Cheddar★/*Cheddar*: hard cow's milk cheese. Dairy product.
Note: do not consume more than approximately ½ oz of cheese three times per week... and never at dinner.

**Cheese★/*Fromage*: food produced thanks to the milk coagulation, the straining of the curds you get and potentially maturing. Dairy product.
Note: do not consume more than approximately ½ oz of cheese three times per week... and never at dinner. Do not consume very fat cheese.

**Cheeseburger/*Cheeseburger*: hamburger with aged cheese.

Cheese gnocchi★★/*Gnocchi au fromage*: ball made of wheat semolina and potatoes enriched with cheese. Carbohydrate.

Cheese ravioli★★/*Ravioli de fromage*: small square of pasta stuffed with various cheese before being poached. Carbohydrate.

Cheese with cereals★/*Fromage aux céréales*: aged cheese with various cereals and/or cereal grains.
Note: do not consume more than approximately ½ oz of cheese three times per week... and never at dinner.

Cheese with dried fruits★/*Fromage aux fruits secs*: aged cheese with various dried fruits.
Note: do not consume more than approximately ½ oz of cheese three times per week... and never at dinner.

Cheese with grains★/*Fromage aux graines*: aged cheese with various grains.
Note: do not consume more than approximately ½ oz of cheese three times per week... and never at dinner.

Cheese with nuts★/*Fromage aux noix*: aged cheese with more or less crushed nuts.
Note: do not consume more than approximately ½ oz of cheese three times per week... and never at dinner.

Cheese with parsley in its rind★/*Fromage à pâte persillée*: blue cheese, fourme d'Ambert, gorgonzola, bleu du Vercors-Sassenage, stilton cheese... Dairy product.
Note: do not consume more than approximately ½ oz of cheese three times per week... and never at dinner.

Cheese with pepper★/*Fromage au poivre*: aged cheese which surface is covered with peppercorns.
Note: do not consume more than approximately ½ oz of cheese three times per week... and never at dinner.

Cherimoya in light syrup - Chestnut flour

Cherimoya in light syrup/*Anone au sirop léger*: poached cherimoya preserved in more or less sugary water. Exotic fruit.

Cherimoya in syrup/*Anone au sirop*: poached cherimoya preserved in very sugary water. Exotic fruit.

Cherry in light syrup/*Cerise au sirop léger*: poached cherry preserved in more or less sugary water.

Cherry in syrup/*Cerise au sirop*: poached cherry preserved in very sugary water.

Cherry juice★/*Jus de cerise*: juice made of the pressing of cherries.

Chervil★★★/*Cerfeuil*: leaf of an aromatic plant used as a condiment. Green vegetable.

Cheshire cheese★/*Chester*: hard cow's milk cheese with raw or pasteurized milk. Dairy product.
Note: do not consume more than approximately ½ oz of cheese three times per week... and never at dinner.

Chestnut★★★/*Châtaigne*: fruit from the sweet chestnut tree, rich in starch. Carbohydrate.

Chestnut cornflakes★★/*Corn flakes de châtaigne*: grilled flakes made of chestnut flour. Carbohydrate. Gluten-free.
Note: do not consume if it's sweetened.

Chestnut cream/*Crème de châtaigne*: chestnut spread.

Chestnut flake★★★/*Flocon de châtaigne*: small portion of dehydrated extruded chestnut. Carbohydrate. Gluten-free.

Chestnut flour★★★/*Farine de châtaigne*: powder made of chestnut milling. Carbohydrate. Gluten-free.

Chestnut milk★★★/*Lait de châtaigne*: plant milk from chestnuts. Lactose-free.
Note: do not consume if it's sweetened.

Chestnut milk cream dessert/*Crème dessert au lait de châtaigne*: vegetable dessert made of chestnut milk, sugar and eggs. Dairy product.

Chestnut pasta★★★/*Pâte alimentaire de châtaigne*: mix to be cooked made of chestnut flour. Carbohydrate. Gluten-free.

Chestnut purée★★★/*Purée de châtaigne*: mashed chestnuts to spread.

Chewing gum★★★/*Chewing-gum*: substance designed to be chewed.
Note: do not consume if it's sweetened.

Chia flour★★★/*Farine de chia*: powder from chia seeds milling. Gluten-free.

Chia seed★★★/*Graine de chia*: chia seed eaten crushed.

Chicken★★★/*Poulet*: baby of the hen, killed before being an adult. Poultry.
Note: cook it without fat: en papillote, in water, grill, roast...

Chicken egg★★★/*Œuf de poule*: edible product from the egg-laying of the chicken.

Chicken ham★★★/*Jambon de poulet*: chicken flesh turned into ham before being cut in thin slices. Cooked meat.

Chicken liver confit/*Confit de foie de volaille*: chicken livers cooked and preserved in their cooking fats.

Chicken nuggets/*Nuggets de poulet*: breaded chicken breast pieces eaten fried.

Chicken rillettes/*Rillettes de poulet*: cooked meat made of chicken meat cooked in its fat.

Chickling vetch: cf. "Lathyrus sativus".

Chickpea★★★/*Pois chiche*: big grey-yellow pea. Carbohydrate. Gluten-free.

Chickpea flake★★★/*Flocon de pois chiches*: small portion of dehydrated chickpea flakes. Carbohydrate. Gluten-free.

Chickpea flour★★★/*Farine de pois chiche*: powder made of chickpea milling. Carbohydrate. Gluten-free.

Chickpea pasta★★★/*Pâte alimentaire de pois chiche*: mix to be cooked made of chickpea flour. Carbohydrate. Gluten-free.

Chicory(1)★★★/*Chicorée(1)*: escarole... Kind of Greek salad. Green vegetable.

Chicory(2)/*Chicorée(2)*: cf. "Chicory coffee".

Chicory coffee★★★/*Café chicorée*: sour chicory with big roots grown as coffee ersatz.
Note: do not consume if it's sweetened.

Chicory seed★★★/*Graine de chicorée*: chicory seed eaten crushed or germinated.

Chili con carne★★/*Chili con carné*: Mexican spicy dish made of kidney beans and ground meat. Red meat.
Note: do not consume more than approximately 4 oz of red meat twice per week.

Chili pepper pâté/Pâte de piment: cf. "Fresh chili pepper".

Chili pepper purée/*Purée de piment*: cf. "Chili pepper".

Chinese artichoke: cf. "Stachys affinis".

Chinese cabbage★★★/*Chou chinois*: kind of two cabbages: Napa cabbage and pak choi.

Chinese noodles of "..."/*Nouille chinoise de "..."*: cf. "Pasta of "..."

Chipolata★/*Chipolata*: thin pork sausage. Cooked meat. *Note: cook it without fat: to grill, to roast, etc.*

Chives★★★/*Ciboulette*: plant from which we eat the hollow and cylindrical leaves.

Chocolate balls/*Crotte de chocolat*: chocolate candy, confection.

Chocolate bar/*Barre chocolatée*: candy made of chocolate and sugar and/or fruits and/or cereals, etc.

Chocolate chip cookie/*Cookie*: small cookie with chocolate, dried fruit, etc. chips.

Chocolate mousse/*Mousse au chocolat*: dessert made of whipped egg whites, chocolate and sugar.

Chocolate spread/*Pâte chocolatée à tartiner*: very sugary and fat mix of chocolate and crushed hazelnuts.

Chokecherry juice★/*Jus de baie d'aronia*: juice made of the pressing of chokecherries.

Chorizo/*Chorizo*: half-dried saucisson seasoned with red chili pepper. Cooked meat.

Choux pastry★/*Pâte à choux*: batter made of butter, flour and eggs.

Chub★★★/*Chevaine*: freshwater fish with white flesh.
Note: cook it without fat: en papillote, in water, grill, roast...

Chuck steak★★/*Paleron de bœuf*: piece of beef to simmer or to boil. Red meat.
Note: do not consume more than approximately 4 oz of red meat twice per week. Cook it without fat: en papillote, in water, grill, roast...

Chufa sedge milk★★★/*Lait de horchata de chufa*: sweetened beverage made from chuff sedge tubers. Lactose-free.
Note: do not consume if it's sweetened.

Chutney/*Chutney*: sweet and sour condiment made of vegetables or fruits cooked with vinegar, spices and sugar.

Cider★/*Cidre*: alcoholic beverage obtained thanks to the apple juice fermentation.
Note: do not drink alcoholic beverage, however no problem if it's cooked.

Cilantro★★★/*Coriandre*: aromatic plant used as a condiment. Green vegetable.

Cilantro seed★★★/*Graine de coriandre*: cilantro seed eaten crushed or germinated.

Cinnamon★★★/*Cannelle*: bark of the cinnamon tree used as seasoning.

Clafoutis/*Clafoutis*: cake baked in the oven made of a mixture of batter, sugar and fruits.

Clam★★★/*Praire*: edible saltwater mollusk.
Note: cook it without fat except with olive oil.

Claytonia perfoliata★★★/*Claytone de Cuba*: vegetable plant you eat as a whole.

Clementine in light syrup/*Clémentine au sirop léger*: poached clementine preserved in more or less sugary water.

Clementine in syrup/*Clémentine au sirop*: poached clementine preserved in very sugary water.

Clementine juice★/*Jus de clémentine*: juice made of the pressing of clementines.

Clove★★★/*Clou de girofle*: fruit from the clove tree used as a spice.

Coalfish★★★/*Goberge*: saltwater fish white white flesh.
Note: cook it without fat: en papillote, in water, grill, roast...

Cochlearia★★★/*Cochléaire*: edible plant which grows in damp places. Green vegetable.

Cockle★★★/*Coque*: edible sea mollusk.
Note: cook it without fat except with olive oil.

Cocktail/*Cocktail*: alcoholic beverage with fruits, fruit juice, syrup, etc.

Cocktail sausage★/*Saucisse cocktail*: small pork sausage with a smoky taste. Cooked meat.
Note: cook it without fat: en papillote, in water, grill...

Cocoa★★/*Cacao*: seed of the cocoa tree used to make chocolate.

Cocoa butter★/*Beurre de cacao*: fat extracted from the cocoa.

Cocoa powder/*Cacao en poudre*: mix of cocoa powder and sugar.

Cocoa powder without sugar★★★/*Cacao en poudre non sucré*: cocoa powder without added sugar.

Coconut - Coconut rock cake

Coconut★★/*Noix de coco*: fruit from the coconut palm. Exotic fruit.

Coconut cream★★★/*Crème de coco*: more or less liquid cream made of coconut milk, substitute to crème fraîche.

Coconut flour★★★/*Farine de coco*: powder from coconut pulp milling. Gluten-free.

Coconut flower sugar★/*Sucre de fleur de coco*: sugar from palm sap. Fast-acting sugar.

Coconut flower syrup/*Sirop de fleur de coco*: sugary syrup made from the palm sap.

Coconut milk★★★/*Lait de coco*: plant milk from coconuts. Lactose-free.
Note: do not consume if it's sweetened.

Coconut milk cream dessert/*Crème dessert au lait de coco*: vegetable dessert made of coconut milk, sugar and eggs. Dairy product.

Coconut milk yogurt★★★/*Yaourt au lait de coco*: coconut milk fermented thanks to lactic acid bacteria, sweetened or not. Dairy product. Lactose-free.
Note: do not consume if it's sweetened.

Coconut oil★★/*Huile de coco*: fatty substance made of coconut.

Coconut powdered sugar★/*Sucre glace de coco*: coconut flower sugar in extremely thin powder. Fast-acting sugar.

Coconut purée★★/*Purée de coco*: mashed coconut pulp to spread.

Coconut rock cake/*Congolais*: small coconut cake.

Coconut water★★★/*Eau de coco*: water from the coconut.

Cocoplum in light syrup/*Icaque au sirop léger*: poached cocoplum preserved in more or less sugary water. Exotic fruit.

Cocoplum in syrup/*Icaque au sirop*: poached cocoplum preserved in very sugary water. Exotic fruit.

Cod★★★/*Morue*: saltwater fish with white flesh.
Note: cook it without fat: en papillote, in water, grill, roast...

Cod liver★★/*Foie de morue*: cod liver in oil sold in can. Offal.

Cod liver oil★★/*Huile de foie de morue*: fatty substance made of cod liver.

Coffee★★★/*Café*: seed of the coffee bush rich in caffeine and drunk once roasted.
Note: do not consume if it's sweetened.

Cognac★/*Cognac*: brandy made of wine from the Cognac area in France.
Note: do not drink alcoholic beverage, however no problem if it's cooked.

Colby cheese★: pasteurised cow's milk cheese. Dairy product.
Note: do not consume more than approximately ½ oz of cheese three times per week... and never at dinner.

Cold-pressed extra virgin olive oil★★/*Huile d'olive extra vierge pressée à froid*: fatty substance made of very high nutritional quality olive.

Coley★★★/*Colin*: saltwater fish with white flesh.
Note: do not consume more than approximately 4 oz of red meat twice per week. Cook it without fat: en papillote, in water, grill, roast...

Colombo★★★/*Colombo*: mix of spices made of garlic, cilantro, chili pepper, cinnamon, turmeric, etc.

Comber★★★/*Serran*: saltwater fish with white flesh.
Note: do not consume more than approximately 4 oz of red meat twice per week. Cook it without fat: en papillote, in water, grill, roast...

Common dace★★★/*Vandoise*: freshwater fish with white flesh.
Note: do not consume more than approximately 4 oz of red meat twice per week. Cook it without fat: en papillote, in water, grill, roast...

Common nase★★★/*Hotu*: freshwater fish with white flesh.
Note: do not consume more than approximately 4 oz of red meat twice per week. Cook it without fat: en papillote, in water, grill, roast...

Common rudd★★★/*Rotengle*: freshwater fish with white flesh.
Note: do not consume more than approximately 4 oz of red meat twice per week. Cook it without fat: en papillote, in water, grill, roast...

Common smooth-hound★★★/*Emissole*: small edible shark with white flesh.
Note: do not consume more than approximately 4 oz of red meat twice per week. Cook it without fat: en papillote, in water, grill, roast...

Compote★★★/*Compotée*: mix of products cooked very slowly.

Comté cheese★/*Comté*: hard cow's milk. Dairy product.
Note: do not consume more than approximately ½ oz of cheese three times per week... and never at dinner.

Concentrate fruit juice★/*Jus de fruit concentré*: reconstituted fruit juice made of fruit juice and water.

Confection/*Confiserie*: various candies.

Confit of duck/*Confit de canard*: duck cooked and preserved in its fat.

Conger★★★/*Congre*: fatty saltwater fish.
Note: do not consume more than approximately 4 oz of red meat twice per week. Cook it without fat: en papillote, in water, grill, roast...

Consommé★★★/*Consommé*: meat stock.

Cooked meat/*Charcuterie*: product made of cooked or raw salted pork meat. See each cooked meat separately.

Cookie without added sugar/*Biscuit sans sucre ajouté*: sweetened cookie without added sugar containing only the sugar that is naturally present in the ingredients. Carbohydrate.

Cooking oil★★/*Huile de friture*: mix of vegetable oils especially made for frying.

Copra oil★★/*Huile de coprah*: fatty substance made of copra.

Coquetdale cheese★: cow's milk cheese with pasteurized milk. Dairy product.
Note: do not consume more than approximately ½ oz of cheese three times per week... and never at dinner.

Coregonus albula - Corn syrup

Coregonus albula★★★/*Corégone*: freshwater fish with white flesh.
Note: cook it without fat: en papillote, in water, grill, roast...

Core oil★★/*Huile de noyaux*: fatty substance made of various fruit cores.

Corn bran★★★/*Son de maïs*: residue of corn milling.

Corn cornflakes★★/*Corn flakes de maïs*: grilled flakes made of sieved corn flakes. Carbohydrate. Gluten-free.
Note: do not consume if it's sweetened.

Corned-beef★★/*Corned beef*: beef meat preserved and salted. Red meat.
Note: do not consume more than approximately 4 oz of red meat twice per week. Cook it without fat: en papillote, in water, grill, roast...

Corn flake★★★/*Flocon de maïs*: small portion of dehydrated corn. Carbohydrate. Gluten-free.

Corn flour★★★/*Farine de maïs*: powder made of not whole-grain corn milling. Carbohydrate. Gluten-free.

Corn oil★★/*Huile de maïs*: fatty substance made of corn.

Corn pasta★★★/*Pâte alimentaire de maïs*: mix to be cooked made of refined corn flour. Carbohydrate. Gluten-free.

Cornstarch★★★/*Fécule de maïs*: not whole-grain corn flour. Carbohydrate.

Corn syrup/*Sirop de maïs*: sweetener made of corn starch.

Cottage cheese★★★: pasteurised cow's milk cheese. Dairy product.
Note: do not consume more than approximately ½ oz of cheese three times per week... and never at dinner.

Cotignac/*Cotignac*: very sugary quince jelly.

Cotton oil★★/*Huile de coton*: fatty substance made of cotton.

Coulis★★★/*Coulis*: sauce made of various food substances transformed into purée.

Coulommiers cheese★/*Coulommiers*: soft cow's milk cheese with bloomy rind. Dairy product.
Note: do not consume more than approximately ½ oz of cheese three times per week... and never at dinner.

Country-style pâté/*Pâté de campagne*: ground meat made of pork meat, fat and poultry livers.

Couscous★★/*Couscous*: North African dish made of hard wheat semolina, meat, fish and various vegetables.

Cowpea★★★/*Dolique*: plant looking like a bean growing in tropical regions. Green vegetable.

Cow's milk cheese★/*Fromage de vache*: cheese made of cow's milk. Dairy product.
Note: do not consume more than approximately ½ oz of cheese three times per week... and never at dinner. Do not consume very fat cheese.

Cow's milk cottage cheese★★★/*Faisselle au lait de vache*: fresh cheese made of cow's milk. Dairy product.
Note: the less fat, the better!

Cow's milk cream dessert/*Crème dessert au lait de vache*: dairy specialty or dessert made of cow's milk, sugar and eggs. Dairy product.

Cow's milk fromage blanc★★★/*Fromage blanc de vache*: fresh cheese made of cow's milk, a bit drained and not aged. Dairy product.
Note: the less fat, the better!

Cow's trotter/*Pied de veau*: veal foot. Offal.

Crab★★★/*Crabe*: sea crustacean you can find on the coastline or in freshwater.
Note: cook it without fat: en papillote, in water...

Crab rillettes★★/*Rillettes de crabe*: cooked meat made of crab flesh cooked in vegetable oil.

Cracker/*Cracker*: small salted cookie for the aperitif. Carbohydrate.

Crambe★★★/*Crambe*: plant also called seakale. Green vegetable.

Cranberry in light syrup/*Canneberge au sirop léger*: poached cranberry preserved in more or less sugary water.

Cranberry in syrup/*Canneberge au sirop*: poached cranberry preserved in very sugary water.

Cranberry juice★/*Jus de cranberry*: juice made of the pressing of cranberries.

Crangon crangon★★★/*Boucaud*: grey shrimp.
Note: cook it without fat or with olive oil.

Crawfish★★★/*Ecrevisse*: freshwater crustacean liked for its flesh.
Note: cook it without fat: en papillote, in water, grill, roast...

Crayfish★★★/*Langouste*: walking crustacean very appreciated for its flesh.
Note: cook it without fat: en papillote, in water, grill, roast...

Crème aux œufs/*Crème aux œufs*: cf. "Cream dessert".

Crème bachique/*Crème bachique*: dessert made of eggs, sugar and rum.

Crème brûlée/*Crème brûlée*: cf. "Cream dessert with cow's milk".

Crème caramel/*Crème renversée*: dessert made of milk, sugar and whisked eggs cooked in a bain-marie and removed from the mold before being turned. Dairy product.

Crepe★★★/*Crêpe*: thin layer of cooked batter made of eggs, milk and flour. Carbohydrate.

Crépinette★/*Crépinette*: flat sausage. Cooked meat.
Note: cook it without fat: grill, roast...

Crimson beebalm★★★/*Monarde écarlate*: plant which leaves are used as an aromatic condiment.

Croissant/*Croissant*: viennoiserie pastry made of flour, butter and sugar.

Croque madame★★/*Croque-madame*: croque-monsieur with an egg on top.

Croque monsieur★★/*Croque-monsieur*: hot dish made of ham and cheese between two slices of sandwich bread.

Crottin de Chavignol★/*Crottin de Chavignol*: small raw goat milk cheese. Dairy product.
Note: do not consume more than approximately ½ oz of cheese three times per week... and never at dinner.

Crouton - Crunchy cassava slice of bread

Crouton★★★/*Croûton*: small piece of fried white bread. Carbohydrate.

Crowdie★★★: pasteurised cow's milk cheese. Dairy product.
Note: do not consume more than approximately ½ oz of cheese three times per week... and never at dinner.

Crucian carp★★★/*Cyprin*: freshwater fish with white flesh.
Note: cook it without fat: en papillote, in water, grill, roast...

Crudité★★★/*Crudité*: green vegetable or fruit eaten raw.

Crumble/*Crumble*: dessert made of fruits covered with sweet shortcrust pastry and baked in the oven.

Crunchy amaranth slice of bread★★/*Tartine craquante amarante*: flat and light extruded slice of bread made of refined amaranth flour. Carbohydrate. Gluten-free.

Crunchy barley slice of bread★★/*Tartine craquante orge*: flat and light extruded slice of bread made of refined barley flour. Carbohydrate.

Crunchy buckwheat slice of bread★★/*Tartine craquante sarrasin*: flat and light extruded slice of bread made of refined buckwheat flour. Carbohydrate. Gluten-free.

Crunchy carob seed slice of bread★★/*Tartine craquante graine de caroube*: flat and light extruded slice of bread made of refined carob seed flour. Carbohydrate. Gluten-free.

Crunchy cassava slice of bread★★/*Tartine craquante manioc*: flat and light extruded slice of bread made of refined cassava flour. Carbohydrate. Gluten-free.

Crunchy chestnut slice of bread★★/*Tartine craquante châtaigne*: flat and light extruded slice of bread made of chestnut flour. Carbohydrate. Gluten-free.

Crunchy chia slice of bread★★/*Tartine craquante chia*: flat and light extruded slice of bread made of chia flour. Carbohydrate. Gluten-free.

Crunchy chickpea slice of bread★★/*Tartine craquante pois chiche*: flat and light extruded slice of bread made of chickpea flour. Carbohydrate. Gluten-free.

Crunchy coconut slice of bread★★/*Tartine craquante coco*: flat and light extruded slice of bread made of coconut flour. Carbohydrate. Gluten-free.

Crunchy corn slice of bread★★/*Tartine craquante maïs*: flat and light extruded slice of bread made of refined corn flour. Carbohydrate. Gluten-free.

Crunchy einkorn wheat slice of bread★★/*Tartine craquante petit épeautre*: flat and light extruded slice of bread made of refined einkorn wheat flour. Carbohydrate.

Crunchy findi slice of bread★★/*Tartine craquante fonio*: flat and light extruded slice of bread made of refined findi flour. Carbohydrate. Gluten-free.

Crunchy flax slice of bread★★/*Tartine craquante lin*: flat and light extruded slice of bread made of flax flour. Carbohydrate. Gluten-free.

Crunchy gluten-free oat slice of bread★★/*Tartine craquante avoine sans gluten*: flat and light extruded slice of bread made of refined and gluten-free oat flour. Carbohydrate.

Crunchy khorasan wheat slice of bread★★/*Tartine craquante kamut*: flat and light extruded slice of bread made of refined khorasan wheat flour. Carbohydrate.

**Crunchy lentil slice of bread
- Crunchy rice slice of bread**

Crunchy lentil slice of bread★★/*Tartine craquante lentille*: flat and light extruded slice of bread made of lentil flour. Carbohydrate. Gluten-free.

Crunchy lupin slice of bread★★/*Tartine craquante lupin*: flat and light extruded slice of bread made of lupin flour. Carbohydrate. Gluten-free.

Crunchy millet slice of bread★★/*Tartine craquante millet*: flat and light extruded slice of bread made of refined millet flour. Carbohydrate. Gluten-free.

Crunchy multi-cereal slice of bread★★★/*Tartine craquante multicéréale*: flat and light extruded slice of bread made of various cereals. Carbohydrate.

Crunchy nutsedge slice of bread★★/*Tartine craquante souchet*: flat and light extruded slice of bread made of nutsedge flour. Carbohydrate. Gluten-free.

Crunchy oat slice of bread★★/*Tartine craquante avoine*: flat and light extruded slice of bread made of refined oat flour. Carbohydrate.

Crunchy onion slice of bread★★/*Tartine craquante oignon*: flat and light extruded slice of bread made of onions. Carbohydrate.

Crunchy peanut slice of bread★★/*Tartine craquante arachide*: flat and light extruded slice of bread made of refined peanut flour. Carbohydrate. Gluten-free.

Crunchy quinoa slice of bread★★/*Tartine craquante quinoa*: flat and light extruded slice of bread made of refined quinoa flour. Carbohydrate. Gluten-free.

Crunchy rice slice of bread★★/*Tartine craquante riz*: flat and light extruded slice of bread made of refined rice flour. Carbohydrate. Gluten-free.

Crunchy rye slice of bread★★/*Tartine craquante seigle*: flat and light extruded slice of bread made of refined rye flour. Carbohydrate.

Crunchy sesame slice of bread★★/*Tartine craquante sésame*: flat and light extruded slice of bread made of sesame. Carbohydrate. Gluten-free.

Crunchy sorghum slice of bread★★/*Tartine craquante sorgho*: flat and light extruded slice of bread made of sorghum flour. Carbohydrate. Gluten-free.

Crunchy soybean slice of bread★★/*Tartine craquante soja*: flat and light extruded slice of bread made of refined soybean flour. Carbohydrate. Gluten-free.

Crunchy spelt slice of bread★★/*Tartine craquante épeautre*: flat and light extruded slice of bread made of refined spelt flour. Carbohydrate.

Crunchy squash seed slice of bread★★/*Tartine craquante pépin de courge*: flat and light extruded slice of bread made of squash seed flour. Carbohydrate. Gluten-free.

Crunchy sweet potato slice of bread★★/*Tartine craquante patate douce*: flat and light extruded slice of bread made of sweet potato flour. Carbohydrate. Gluten-free.

Crunchy teff slice of bread★★/*Tartine craquante teff*: flat and light extruded slice of bread made of refined teff flour. Carbohydrate. Gluten-free.

Crunchy wheat slice of bread★★/*Tartine craquante froment*: flat and light extruded slice of bread made of refined tender wheat flour. Carbohydrate.

**Crunchy whole-grain amaranth slice of bread
- Crunchy whole-grain oat slice of bread**

Crunchy whole-grain amaranth slice of bread★★/*Tartine craquante amarante complète*: flat and light extruded slice of bread made of whole-grain amaranth flour. Carbohydrate. Gluten-free.

Crunchy whole-grain barley slice of bread★★/*Tartine craquante orge complète*: flat and light extruded slice of bread made of whole-grain barley flour. Carbohydrate.

Crunchy whole-grain buckwheat slice of bread★★/*Tartine craquante sarrasin complète*: flat and light extruded slice of bread made of whole-grain buckwheat flour. Carbohydrate. Gluten-free.

Crunchy whole-grain corn slice of bread★★/*Tartine craquante maïs complète*: flat and light extruded slice of bread made of whole-grain corn flour. Carbohydrate. Gluten-free.

Crunchy whole-grain einkorn wheat slice of bread★★/*Tartine craquante petit épeautre complète*: flat and light extruded slice of bread made of whole-grain einkorn wheat flour. Carbohydrate.

Crunchy whole-grain findi slice of bread★★/*Tartine craquante fonio complète*: flat and light extruded slice of bread made of whole-grain findi flour. Carbohydrate. Gluten-free.

Crunchy whole-grain khorasan wheat slice of bread★★/*Tartine craquante kamut complète*: flat and light extruded slice of bread made of whole-grain khorasan wheat flour. Carbohydrate.

Crunchy whole-grain oat slice of bread★★/*Tartine craquante avoine complète*: flat and light extruded slice of bread made of whole-grain oat flour. Carbohydrate.

Crunchy whole-grain peanut slice of bread★★/*Tartine craquante arachide complète*: flat and light extruded slice of bread made of whole-grain peanut flour. Carbohydrate. Gluten-free.

Crunchy whole-grain quinoa slice of bread★★/*Tartine craquante quinoa complète*: flat and light extruded slice of bread made of whole-grain quinoa. Carbohydrate. Gluten-free.

Crunchy whole-grain rice slice of bread★★/*Tartine craquante riz complet*: flat and light extruded slice of bread made of whole-grain rice flour. Carbohydrate. Gluten-free.

Crunchy whole-grain rye slice of bread★★/*Tartine craquante seigle complète*: flat and light extruded slice of bread made of whole-grain rye flour. Carbohydrate.

Crunchy whole-grain soybean slice of bread★★/*Tartine craquante soja complète*: flat and light extruded slice of bread made of whole-grain soybean flour. Carbohydrate. Gluten-free.

Crunchy whole-grain spelt slice of bread★★/*Tartine craquante épeautre complète*: flat and light extruded slice of bread made of whole-grain spelt flour. Carbohydrate.

Crunchy whole-grain teff slice of bread★★/*Tartine craquante teff complète*: flat and light extruded slice of bread made of whole-grain teff flour. Carbohydrate. Gluten-free.

Crunchy wholewheat slice of bread★★/*Tartine craquante blé complète*: flat and light extruded slice of bread made of wholewheat flour. Carbohydrate.

Crunchy yam slice of bread★★/*Tartine craquante igname*: flat and light extruded slice of bread made of refined yam flour. Carbohydrate. Gluten-free.

Crushed spelt/*Epeautre concassé*: cf. "Spelt bulgur".

Crustacean/*Crustacé*: crab, lobster, shrimp, etc. (See each crustacean separately).

Cube of beef broth★★★/*Bouillon de bœuf en cube*: cube of dehydrated industrial beef broth.

Cube of beef stew broth/*Bouillon de pot-au-feu en cube*: cf. "Cube of beef broth".

Cube of chicken broth★★★/*Bouillon de volaille en cube*: cube of dehydrated industrial chicken broth.

Cube of low-fat beef broth★★★/*Bouillon de bœuf dégraissé en cube*: cube of low-fat and dehydrated industrial beef broth.

Cube of low-fat chicken broth★★★/*Bouillon de volaille dégraissé en cube*: cube of low-fat and dehydrated industrial chicken broth.

Cube of low-fat vegetable broth★★★/*Bouillon de légumes dégraissé en cube*: cube of low-fat and dehydrated industrial vegetable broth.

Cube of low-salt chicken broth★★★/*Bouillon de volaille allégé en sel en cube*: cube of light-sodium and dehydrated industrial chicken broth.

Cube of salt-free vegetable broth★★★/*Bouillon de légumes sans sel en cube*: cube of salt-free and dehydrated industrial vegetable broth.

Cube of vegetable broth★★★/*Bouillon de légumes en cube*: cube of dehydrated industrial vegetable broth.

Cucumber★★★/*Concombre*: vegetable plant grown for its long fruit.

Cuidité★★★/*Cuidité*: green vegetable or fruit eaten cooked.

Cumin★★★/*Cumin*: spice.

Cumin seed★★★/*Graine de cumin*: cumin seed eaten crushed or germinated.

Cup cheese★: melted cheese. Dairy product.
Note: do not consume more than approximately ½ oz of cheese three times per week... and never at dinner.

Curaçao/*Curaçao*: liqueur made of orange peel, sugar and eau de vie.

Curly endive (lettuce)★★★/*Frisée (laitue)*: lettuce with curly leaves eaten in salad. Green vegetable.

Curry★★★/*Curry*: mix of Indian spices.

Curuba★★/*Curuba*: exotic fruit from Asia.

Custard(1)/*Crème anglaise*: cream with a base thickened on the heat and flavored with vanilla. Dairy product.

Custard(2)/*Crème pâtissière*: cream made of flour, eggs, milk and sugar. Dairy product.

Custard apple★★/*Chérimole*: fruit from the cherimoya. Exotic fruit.
Note: consume it in moderation, immediately after the meal.

Cuttlefish★★★/*Seiche*: saltwater mollusk close to the squid.
Note: cook it without fat: en papillote, in water, grill, roast...

Cyclanthera★★★/*Cyclanthère*: young fruit preserved in vinegar.

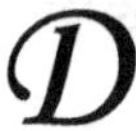

Dab★★★/***Limande***: flat saltwater fish with white flesh.
Note: cook it without fat: en papillote, in water, grill, roast...

Dandelion★★★/***Pissenlit***: plant from which we eat the young leaves in salad. Green vegetable.

Dandelion coffee★★★/***Café de pissenlit***: drink made of dried dandelion roots.
Note: do not consume if it's sweetened.

Dark chocolate★/***Chocolat noir***: chocolate containing between 43 % and 100 % of cocoa and cocoa butter, the rest being mainly sugar.

Date honey/*Sirop de datte***: sugary syrup made of date extracts.

Date jelly/*Pâte de datte***: cf. "Dried date".

Daube★★/***Daube***: culinary technique consisting in braising beef with a base of red wine. Red meat.
Note: do not consume more than approximately 4 oz of red meat twice per week.

Dauphinois (gratin)★★/***Dauphinois (gratin)***: dish made of thin slices of grilled potatoes with milk, butter and cheese.

Decaffeinated coffee★★★/***Café soluble décaféiné***: grains of dehydrated decaffeinated coffee.
Note: do not consume if it's sweetened.

Decaffeinated espresso★★★/***Expresso décaféiné***: caffeine-free express coffee.
Note: do not consume if it's sweetened.

Deer (meat)★ ★/*Daim (viande de)*: game from which we eat the meat. Red meat.
Note: do not consume more than approximately 4 oz of red meat twice per week. Cook it without fat: en papillote, in water, grill, roast...

Dehydrated green vegetable soup★★★/*Potage de légumes verts déshydraté*: dehydrated industrial soup.

Derby cheese★: raw or pasteurised cow's milk cheese. Dairy product.
Note: do not consume more than approximately ½ oz of cheese three times per week... and never at dinner.

Dessert/*Entremets*: sugary dish which is not pastry. Dairy product.

Dessert wine/*Vin liquoreux*: white wine which contains more than 45 grams of sugar per liter.

Deviled egg★/*Œuf mimosa*: egg cut in half, the egg yolk is removed and mixed with mayonnaise, before filling the hole in the white part of the egg with this mixture.

"Diet" extruded cereal★/*Céréale extrudée "de régime"*: sugar-free and low-calorie swelled cereal. High glycemic index. Carbohydrate.
Note: do not consume if it's sweetened.

"Diet" salt★★★/*Sel "de régime"*: potassium chloride used to season dishes. Some diet salts offer one third of the total quantity of sodium chloride (standard table salt).

Dill★★★/*Aneth*: aromatic umbellifer plant.

Dock★★★/*Patience*: vegetable plant from which we eat the leaves. Green vegetable.

Doe (meat)★★/*Biche (viande de)*: female deer. Red meat. Game.
Note: do not consume more than approximately 4 oz of red meat twice per week. Cook it without fat: en papillote, in water, grill, roast...

Dog cockle★★★/*Amande marin*: edible sea mollusk.
Note: cook it without fat or with olive oil.

Dogfish★★★/*Roussette*: cartilaginous saltwater fish (small shark) with white flesh.
Note: cook it without fat: en papillote, in water, grill, roast...

Donax★★★/*Donax*: small edible sea mollusk.
Note: cook it without fat or with olive oil.

Dorset blue vinney★: raw cow's milk cheese. Dairy product.
Note: do not consume more than approximately ½ oz of cheese three times per week... and never at dinner.

Double cream cheese★/*Fromage double crème*: cheese containing between 60 and 75% of fats. Dairy product.
Note: do not consume more than approximately ½ oz of cheese three times per week... and never at dinner.

Dovedale cheese★: pasteurised cow's milk cheese. Dairy product.
Note: do not consume more than approximately ½ oz of cheese three times per week... and never at dinner.

Double Gloucester★: raw or pasteurised cow's milk cheese. Dairy product.
Note: do not consume more than approximately ½ oz of cheese three times per week... and never at dinner.

Dried apple★★/*Pomme séchée*: apple which went under a desiccation process under the sun.

Dried apricot/*Abricot sec*: fresh apricot dehydrated thanks to the action of the sun or that of the heat.

Dried aronia/*Aronia séchée*: aronia which went under a desiccation process under the sun.

Dried azerole/*Azerole séchée*: azerole which went under a desiccation process under the sun.

Dried banana/*Banane séchée*: banana which went under a desiccation process. Exotic fruit.

Dried bean★★★/*Haricot sec*: bean seed eaten ripe such as split peas, beans from Soissons, cranberry beans, navy beans, kidney beans, pinto beans, black turtle beans, lentils, chickpeas, flageolets, etc. Carbohydrate.

Dried blackberry/*Mûre séchée*: blackberry which went under a desiccation process under the sun.

Dried blackcurrant/*Cassis séché*: blackcurrant which went under a desiccation process under the sun.

Dried button mangosteen/*Mangoustan séché*: button mangosteen which went under a desiccation process under the sun. Exotic fruit.

Dried carambola/*Carambole séchée*: carambola which went under a desiccation process under the sun. Exotic fruit.

Dried cherimoya/*Anone séchée*: cherimoya which went under a desiccation process under the sun. Exotic fruit.

Dried cherry/*Cerise séchée*: cherry which went under a desiccation process under the sun.

Dried chili pepper★★★/*Piment sec*: chili pepper which went under a desiccation process under the sun. Green vegetable.

Dried clementine/*Clémentine séchée*: clementine which went under a desiccation process under the sun.

Dried coconut★★/*Noix de coco séchée*: coconut pulp fragment eaten after being completely desiccated. Exotic fruit.

Dried cranberry/*Canneberge séchée*: cranberry which went under a desiccation process under the sun.

Dried date/*Datte séchée*: fruit from the date palm which dried under the sun. Exotic fruit.

Dried fatty fish★★★/*Poisson gras séché*: fatty fish which went under a desiccation process.

Dried fig/*Figue séchée*: fig which has been dried under the sun

Dried fruit/*Fruit sec*: fruit which went under a desiccation process under the sun. See each of them depending on their own name.

Dried fruits breakfast cookie/*Biscuit pour petit-déjeuner aux fruits secs*: cookie with dried fruits adapted to breakfast. Carbohydrate.

Dried goji berry/*Baie de goji séchée*: small red fruit eaten after a complete desiccation process.

Dried grapefruit/*Pamplemousse séché*: grapefruit which went under a desiccation process under the sun.

Dried guava/*Goyave séchée*: guava which went under a desiccation process under the sun. Exotic fruit.

Dried jackfruit/*Jaque séché*: jackfruit which went under a desiccation process under the sun.

Dried jujube/*Jujube séchée*: jujube which went under a desiccation process under the sun. Exotic fruit.

Dried kaki/*Kaki séché*: kaki which went under a desiccation process under the sun.

Dried kiwi/*Kiwi séché*: kiwi which went under a desiccation process under the sun.

Dried kumquat/*Kumquat séché*: kumquat which went under a desiccation process under the sun.

Dried lean fish★★★/*Poisson maigre séché*: lean fish which went under a desiccation process.

Dried legume★★★/*Légume sec*: legume seeds (lentils, navy beans, beans from Soissons, cranberry beans, favas, chickpeas, split peas, kidney beans, black turtle beans, lupins, mojette beans, common vetches, etc.) eaten ripe. Carbohydrate.

Dried lemon★★★/*Citron séché*: lemon which went under a desiccation process under the sun.
Note: consume it in moderation, immediately after the meal.

Dried longan/*Longane séchée*: longan which went under a desiccation process under the sun. Exotic fruit.

Dried lychee/*Litchi séché*: lychee which went under a desiccation process under the sun. Exotic fruit.

Dried Malay rose apple/*Jambose séchée*: Malay rose apple which went under a desiccation process under the sun. Exotic fruit.

Dried mandarin/*Mandarine séchée*: mandarin which went under a desiccation process under the sun.

Dried mango/*Mangue séchée*: mango which went under a desiccation process under the sun. Exotic fruit.

Dried medlar/*Nèfle séchée*: medlar which went under a desiccation process under the sun.

Dried melon/*Melon séché*: melon which went under a desiccation process under the sun.

Dried mirabelle plum/*Mirabelle séchée*: mirabelle plum which went under a desiccation process under the sun.

Dried mombins/*Mombin séché*: mombins which went under a desiccation process under the sun. Exotic fruit.

Dried mulberries/*Mulberries séchée*: mulberries which went under a desiccation process under the sun.

Dried mushroom★★★/*Champignon séché*: fresh mushroom which went under a desiccation process. Green vegetable.

Dried myrciaria/*Camu-camu séchée*: myrciaria which went under a desiccation process under the sun. Exotic fruit.

Dried orange/*Orange séchée*: orange which went under a desiccation process under the sun.

Dried papaya/*Papaye séchée*: papaya which went under a desiccation process under the sun. Exotic fruit.

Dried passion fruit/*Fruit de la passion séché*: passion fruit which went under a desiccation process.

Dried peach/*Pêche séchée*: peach which went under a desiccation process under the sun.

Dried pear/*Poire séchée*: pear which went under a desiccation process under the sun.

Dried physalis/*Physalis séchée*: physalis which went under a desiccation process under the sun. Exotic fruit.

Dried pineapple/*Ananas séché*: pineapple which went under a desiccation process under the sun. Exotic fruit.

Dried pitaya/*Pitaya séchée*: pitaya which went under a desiccation process under the sun. Exotic fruit.

Dried pomegranate/*Grenade séchée*: pomegranate which went under a desiccation process under the sun. Exotic fruit.

Dried quince/*Coing séché*: quince which went under a desiccation process.

Dried rambutan/*Ramboutan séché*: rambutan which went under a desiccation process under the sun. Exotic fruit.

Dried raspberry/*Framboise séchée*: fresh raspberry which went under a desiccation process.

Dried redcurrant/*Groseille séchée*: redcurrant which went under a desiccation process under the sun.

Dried sapodilla fruit/Sapotille séchée: sapodilla fruit which went under a desiccation process under the sun. Exotic fruit.

Dried sloe/*Prunelle séchée*: sloe which went under a desiccation process under the sun.

Dried strawberry/*Fraise séchée*: fresh strawberry which went under a desiccation process.

Dried tamarind fruit/*Tamarin séché*: tamarind fruit which went under a desiccation process under the sun. Exotic fruit.

Dried watermelon/*Pastèque séchée*: watermelon which went under a desiccation process under the sun.

Dry-cured ham★★★/*Jambon sec*: raw pork ham salted before being dried. Cooked meat.

Duck★★★/*Canard*: edible palmiped bird. Poultry.
Note: cook it without fat: en papillote, in water, grill, roast...

Duck egg★★★/*Œuf de cane*: edible product from the egg-laying of the female duck.

Duck fat/*Graisse de canard*: duck fat used to make confits.

Duck liver pâté/*Pâté de foie de canard*: minced duck liver cooked before being put in a baking pan. Cooked meat.

Dulse★★★/*Dulce*: edible red seaweed.

Dunlop cheese★: raw or pasteurised cow's milk cheese. Dairy product.
Note: do not consume more than approximately ½ oz of cheese three times per week... and never at dinner.

Durio zibethinus★★/*Durian*: exotic fruit from Asia.

Duxelles★★★/*Duxelles*: minced mixture of mushrooms, onions and shallots.

E

Ear of corn★★★/*Epi de maïs*: young corn shoot considered as a green vegetable.

Eau de vie★/*Eau-de-vie*: alcohol beverage made thanks to a distillation process.
Note: do not drink alcoholic beverage, however no problem if it's cooked.

Edam cheese★/*Edam*: semi-hard cheese with raw cow's milk. Dairy product.
Note: do not consume more than approximately ½ oz of cheese three times per week... and never at dinner.

Edible cortinarius★★★/*Cortinaire comestible*: wild mushroom. Green vegetable.

Edible flower★★★/*Fleur comestible*: flower used as a decoration for a dish and perfectly edible.

Edible mushroom (wild or grown) ★★★/*Champignon comestible (sauvage ou cultivé)*: no-chlorophyll cryptogam. Only a few hundreds of them out of more than 50000 are edible. Green vegetable.

Edible nutsedge★★★/*Souchet comestible*: plant from which we eat the tubers. Green vegetable.

Eel★★★/*Anguille*: fatty freshwater fish.
Note: cook it without fat: en papillote, in water, grill, roast...

Eggnog/*Lait de poule*: sweetened beverage made thanks to the mixing of a chicken egg yolk in a glass of milk.

Eggplant★★★/*Aubergine*: annual vegetable plant especially grown in Mediterranean regions. Green vegetable.

Egg white★★★/*Blanc d'œuf*: edible part of the egg without the egg yolk.

Egg yolk★★/*Jaune d'œuf*: yellow part of the egg.

Einkorn bulgur★★★/*Boulgour de petit épeautre*: sieved and crushed einkorn steamed or cooked in water. Carbohydrate.

Einkorn wheat flake★★★/*Flocon de petit-épeautre*: small portion of dehydrated einkorn wheat. Carbohydrate.

Einkorn wheat pasta★★★/*Pâte alimentaire de petit épeautre*: mix to be cooked made of refined einkorn wheat flour. Carbohydrate.

Emmental cheese★/*Emmental*: hard cow's milk cheese. Dairy product.
Note: do not consume more than approximately ½ oz of cheese three times per week... and never at dinner.

Emperor fish★★★/*Capitaine*: saltwater fish with white flesh.
Note: cook it without fat: en papillote, in water, grill, roast...

Endive★★★/*Endive*: excessive bud which we eat in salad or as a vegetable. Green vegetable.

Energy drink/*Boisson énergisante*: fizzy or still drink made of taurine and caffeine.

English sauce★★/*Sauce anglaise*: white sauce with chicken stock, Madeira wine and tomato purée.

Epoisses de Bourgogne★/*Epoisses*: soft cow's milk cheese with washed rind. Dairy product.
Note: do not consume more than approximately ½ oz of cheese three times per week... and never at dinner.

Escarole★★★/*Scarole*: curly endive with large leaves eaten in salad. Green vegetable.

Espresso★★★/*Expresso*: express coffee rich in caffeine.
Note: do not consume if it's sweetened.

Eurasian minnow★★★/*Vairon*: small freshwater fish with white flesh.
Note: cook it without fat.

European barracuda★★★/*Spet*: saltwater fish with white flesh.
Note: cook it without fat: en papillote, in water, grill, roast...

European sprat★★★/*Sprat*: fatty saltwater fish.
Note: cook it without fat: en papillote, in water, grill, roast...

Exotic fruit/*Fruit exotique*: fruit coming from far away foreign countries. See each of them depending on their own name.

Eye of round★★/*Noix de bœuf*: piece of beef to roast. Red meat.
Note: do not consume more than approximately 4 oz of red meat twice per week. Cook it without fat: en papillote, in water, grill, roast...

F

Fajita★★★/*Fajita*: corn tortilla. Carbohydrate. Gluten-free.

Falafel★★★/*Falafel*: small fava bean and chickpea doughnut-shaped patty. Carbohydrate. Gluten-free.

Farmhouse bread★★★/*Pain de campagne*: bread with a thick crust made of leaven and wheat flour milled on a millstone. Carbohydrate.

Fast/*Jeûne*: deprivation of food for a more or less long period of time.

Fatback/*Lard*: adipose piece of the pork.

Fatty fish - 15% fat lightly salted butter

Fatty fish★★★/*Poisson gras*: fish with brown flesh, rich in omega 3 and in polyunsaturated fats: mackerel, sardine, tuna, herring, trout, char, salmon, anchovy, eel, conger, etc.
Note: cook it without fat: en papillote, in water, grill, roast...

Fatty fish fillet★★★/*Filet de poisson gras*: slice of fatty fish in general without fishbone.
Note: cook it without fat: in water, grill, roast...

Fatty slice★★/*Tranche grasse*: piece of beef to grill. Red meat.
Note: do not consume more than approximately 4 oz of red meat twice per week. Cook it without fat: en papillote, in water, grill, roast...

Fava bean★★★/*Fève*: seed from a vegetable annual plant. Carbohydrate.

Fennel★★★/*Fenouil*: vegetable and aromatic plant from which we eat the plump leafstalk base. Green vegetable.

Fennel seed★★★/*Graine de fenouil*: fennel seed eaten crushed or germinated.

Fenugreek seed★★★/*Graine de fenugrec*: fenugreek seed eaten crushed or germinated.

15% fat ground beef steak★★/*Steak haché de bœuf à 15% de matières grasses*: ground beef meat containing 15% of fat. To grill.
Note: do not consume more than approximately 4 oz of red meat twice per week. Cook it without fat: en papillote, in water, grill, roast...

15% fat lightly salted butter★★/*Beurre demi-sel à 15% de matières grasses*: lightly salted butter which fat quantity has been reduced from more than three fourths compared to traditional butter.
Note: consume it in moderation. Do not cook with it.

15% fat lightly unsalted butter★★/*Beurre doux à 15% de matières grasses*: unsalted butter which fat quantity has been reduced from more than three fourths compared to traditional butter.
Note: consume it in moderation. Do not cook with it.

Fig jelly/*Pâte de figue*: cf. "Dried fig".

Fillet (beef meat)★★/*Filet (viande de bœuf)*: tender and plump piece of beef. Red meat.
Note: do not consume more than approximately 4 oz of red meat twice per week. Cook it without fat: en papillote, in water, grill, roast...

Fillet (lamb meat)★★/*Filet (viande d'agneau)*: tender and plump piece of lamb. Red meat.
Note: do not consume more than approximately 4 oz of red meat twice per week. Cook it without fat: en papillote, in water, grill, roast...

Fillet of duck breast★★/*Magret*: fillet of duck flesh. Red meat.
Note: do not consume more than approximately 4 oz of red meat twice per week. Cook it without fat: en papillote, in water, grill, roast...

Fillet (pork meat)★★★/*Filet (viande de porc)*: tender and plump piece of pork.
Note: cook it without fat: en papillote, in water, grill, roast...

Fillet (veal meat)★★★/*Filet (viande de veau)*: tender and plump piece of veal.
Note: cook it without fat: en papillote, in water, grill, roast...

Financier★★★/*Financière*: side dish or sauce made of mushrooms, truffles, sweetbread, etc.

Findi pasta - Flan (mixture)

Findi pasta★★★/*Pâte alimentaire de fonio*: mix to be cooked made of refined findi flour. Carbohydrate. Gluten-free.

Fish pâté en croûte★★/*Pâté de poisson en croûte*: dish made of ground fish wrapped in puff pastry.

Fish stock★★★/*Fumet de poisson*: very reduced stock made of fish.

Fish terrine★/*Pain de poisson*: dish made of potatoes, fish, butter and eggs and served cold with a mayonnaise.
Note: do not consume mayonnaise.

5% fat ground beef steak★★★/*Steak haché de bœuf à 5% de matières grasses*: ground beef meat containing 5% of fat. To grill.
Note: do not consume more than approximately 4 oz of red meat twice per week. Cook it without fat: grill, roast...

5% fat lightly salted butter★★★/*Beurre demi-sel à 5% de matières grasses*: lightly salted butter which fat quantity is very low compared to traditional butter.

5% fat lightly unsalted butter★★★/*Beurre doux à 5% de matières grasses*: unsalted butter which fat quantity is very low compared to traditional butter.

Fizzy water★★★/*Eau gazeuse*: natural water enriched or naturally rich in carbon dioxide.

Flageolet★★★/*Flageolet*: seed from a vegetable legume. Carbohydrate.

Flan (mixture)★★/*Flan (appareil à)*: mixture made of eggs, milk, crème fraîche, with or without flour, salted or sweet, to which ingredients (green vegetables, fish, meat, etc.) are added or not.
Note: do not consume if it's sweetened.

Flank (beef)★★/*Flanchet (de bœuf)*: beef meat. Red meat.
Note: do not consume more than approximately 4 oz of red meat twice per week. Cook it without fat: en papillote, in water, grill, roast...

Flank steak★★/*Bavette*: tender piece of beef. Red meat.
Note: do not consume more than approximately 4 oz of red meat twice per week. Cook it without fat: en papillote, in water, grill, roast...

Flank (veal)★★★/*Flanchet (de veau)*: veal meat.
Note: cook it without fat: en papillote, in water, grill...

Flavored yogurt/*Yaourt aromatisé*: goat, sheep or cow's milk fermented thanks to lactic acid bacteria before being sweetened and flavored. Dairy product.

Flax flour★★★/*Farine de lin*: powder made of flax milling. Carbohydrate. Gluten-free.

Flax pasta★★★/*Pâte alimentaire de lin*: mix to be cooked made of flax flour. Carbohydrate. Gluten-free.

Flaxseed★★★/*Graine de lin*: flax seed eaten crushed.

Floating island/*Ile flottante*: caramelized beaten egg white put on custard with grilled almonds.

Flounder★★★/*Flet*: flat saltwater fish with white flesh.
Note: cook it without fat: en papillote, in water, grill...

Foie gras/Foie gras: liver which is the result of goose or duck force-feeding. Cooked meat.

Foil or baking parchment parcel★★★/*En papillote*: aluminium sheet used to wrap some foods, usually fresh fish, to steam them or to bake them in the oven without adding any fat.

Fondue/*Fondue*: dish made of Emmental cheese and gruyère strips melted in white wine.

Fonio flour★★★/*Farine de fonio*: powder made of not whole-grain folio milling. Carbohydrate. Gluten-free.

Fontainebleau cheese★/*Fontainebleau*: cow's milk fromage frais. Dairy product.
Note: do not consume more than approximately ½ oz of cheese three times per week... and never at dinner.

Fontina★/*Fontine*: raw cow's milk semi-hard cheese. Dairy product.
Note: do not consume more than approximately ½ oz of cheese three times per week... and never at dinner.

41% fat lightly salted butter★★/*Beurre demi-sel à 41% de matières grasses*: lightly salted butter which fat quantity is half the quantity of traditional butter.
Note: consume it in moderation. Do not cook with it.

41% fat lightly unsalted butter★★/*Beurre doux à 41% de matières grasses*: unsalted butter which fat quantity is half the quantity of traditional butter.
Note: consume it in moderation. Do not cook with it.

Fourme★/*Fourme*: cow's milk cheese. Dairy product.
Note: do not consume more than approximately ½ oz of cheese three times per week... and never at dinner.

Foutou★★★/*Foutou*: yam flour cooked in water and served under the shape of a ball. Gluten-free.

Frangipane cream/*Crème frangipane*: custard with almond powder. Dairy product.

French fries★/*Frites*: fried potatoes. Carbohydrate. Gluten-free.

French toast/*Pain perdu*: dessert made of stale bread or brioche soaked in milk and in eggs, sweetened and fried. Carbohydrate.

Fresh apple★★★/*Pomme fraîche*: edible fruit from the apple tree.

Fresh apricot★★/*Abricot frais*: fresh fruit from the apricot tree.

Fresh aronia★★/*Aronia fraîche*: little red or black berry. Red fruit.

Fresh azerole★★/*Azerole fraîche*: small red fruit looking like a cherry, very rich in vitamin C.

Fresh blackberry★★/*Mûre fraîche*: edible fruit from the blackberry bush.

Fresh blackcurrant★★/*Cassis frais*: fruit, small black berry.

Fresh button mangosteen★★/*Mangoustan frais*: fruit from the mangosteen. Exotic fruit.

Fresh carambola★★/*Carambole fraîche*: fruit with juicy and acid flesh. Exotic fruit.

Fresh cherimoya★★/*Anone fraîche*: edible tropical fruit. Exotic fruit.

Fresh cherry★★/*Cerise fraîche*: fruit from the cherry tree.

Fresh chili pepper★★★/*Piment frais*: vegetable plant from which we eat the fruit which is more or less spicy. Green vegetable.

Fresh clementine★★/*Clémentine fraîche*: fruit from the clementine tree.

Fresh cocoplum - Fresh jujube

Fresh cocoplum★★/*Icaque fraîche*: edible fruit from the chrysobalanus icaco. Exotic fruit.

Fresh cranberry★★/*Canneberge fraîche*: red berry looking like a vaccinium. Red fruit.

Fresh date★★/*Datte fraîche*: fruit from the date palm. Exotic fruit.

Fresh fig★★/*Figue fraîche*: fresh fruit from the fig tree.

Fresh fruit/*Fruit frais*: apple, pear, banana, etc. See each of them depending on their own name.

Fresh fruit salad★★/*Salade de fruits frais*: mix of various fresh fruits without adding anything.

Fresh goji berry★★/*Baie de goji fraîche*: small red berry from a Chinese bush.

Fresh grape★★/*Raisin frais*: fruit from the vine.

Fresh grapefruit★★/*Pamplemousse frais*: edible fruit from the grapefruit tree.

Fresh green vegetable preserved after being cooked★★★/*Légume vert frais cuisiné en conserve*: fresh green vegetable treated in various industrial ways before being put in cans.

Fresh green vegetable preserved without being cooked★★★/*Légume vert frais en conserve non cuisiné*: fresh green vegetable, blanched before being preserved in brine and put in cans.

Fresh guava★★/*Goyave fraîche*: fruit from the common guava. Exotic fruit.

Fresh jujube★★/*Jujube fraîche*: fruit from the ziziphus. Exotic fruit.

Fresh kaki★★/*Kaki frais*: fruit from the date plum tree.

Fresh kiwi★★/*Kiwi frais*: fruit from the actinidia.

Fresh kumquat★★/*Kumquat frais*: fruit from the kumquat, yellow citrus fruit.

Fresh lemon★★★/*Citron frais*: fruit from the lemon tree.

Fresh longan★★/*Longane fraîche*: fruit from the longan tree. Exotic fruit.

Fresh lychee★★/*Litchi frais*: fruit from the lychee. Exotic fruit.

Fresh mackerel★★★/*Maquereau frais*: fatty saltwater fish freshly caught.
Note: cook it without fat: en papillote, in water, grill, roast...

Fresh malay rose apple★★/*Jambose fraîche*: fruit from the syzygium malaccense. Exotic fruit.

Fresh mandarin★★/*Mandarine fraîche*: fruit from the mandarin tree.

Fresh mango★★/*Mangue fraîche*: fruit from the mango tree. Exotic fruit.

Fresh medlar★★/*Nèfle fraîche*: fruit from the medlar tree eaten overripe.

Fresh melon★★/*Melon frais*: fruit from the cucurbits family.

Fresh mirabelle plum★★/*Mirabelle fraîche*: small yellow plum.

Fresh mombins★★/*Mombin frais*: fruit from spondias. Exotic fruit.

Fresh mulberries★★/*Mulberries fraîche*: small berry very similar to the blackberry but longer.

Fresh myrciaria★★/*Camu-camu fraîche*: red orangey fruit looking like a plum and rich in vitamin C. Exotic fruit.

Fresh nectarine★★/*Brugnon frais*: fruit from the nectarine tree.

Fresh orange★★/*Orange fraîche*: fruit from the orange tree.

Fresh papaya★★/*Papaye fraîche*: fruit from the papaya tree. Exotic fruit.

Fresh passion fruit★★/*Fruit de la passion frais*: fruit from some varieties of passion vine. Exotic fruit.

Fresh peach★★/*Pêche fraîche*: edible fruit from the peach tree.

Fresh pear★★/*Poire fraîche*: fruit from the pear tree.

Fresh physalis★★/*Physalis fraîche*: small round fruit. Exotic fruit.

Fresh pineapple★★/*Ananas frais*: big tropical fruit with sugary and tasty flesh. Exotic fruit.

Fresh pitaya★★/*Pitaya fraîche*: exotic fruit also called dragon fruit.

Fresh plum★★/*Prune fraîche*: fruit from the plum tree.

Fresh pomegranate★★/*Grenade fraîche*: fruit from the pomegranate tree. Exotic fruit.

Fresh quince★★/*Coing frais*: yellow fruit from the quince tree.

Fresh rambutan★★/*Ramboutan frais*: fruit from the rambutan. Exotic fruit.

Fresh raspberry★★/*Framboise fraîche*: fresh fruit from the raspberry bush.

Fresh redcurrant★★/*Groseille fraîche*: edible fruit from the currant bush.

Fresh salak★★/*Salacca frais*: fruit from a palm family, exotic fruit.

Fresh salmon★★★/*Saumon frais*: fatty fish found in freshwater.
Note: cook it without fat: en papillote, in water, grill, roast...

Fresh sapodilla fruit★★/*Sapotille fraîche*: fruit from the sapodilla. Exotic fruit.

Fresh sardine★★★/*Sardine fraîche*: fatty saltwater fish freshly caught.
Note: cook it without fat: en papillote, in water, grill, roast...

Fresh sloe★★/*Prunelle fraîche*: fruit from the sloe tree.

Fresh sorb★★/*Sorbe fraîche*: fruit from the sorb tree.

Fresh strawberry★★★/*Fraise fraîche*: plump fruit from the strawberry plant.

Fresh tamarind fruit★★/*Tamarin frais*: fruit from the tamarind. Laxative exotic fruit.

Fresh tuna★★★/*Thon frais*: fatty saltwater fish freshly caught.
Note: cook it without fat: en papillote, in water, grill, roast...

**Freshwater fish
- Fruit compote with no added sugar**

Freshwater fish★★★/*Poisson de rivière*: every fatty and lean fish found in rivers.
Note: cook it without fat: en papillote, in water, grill, roast...

Fresh watermelon★★★/*Pastèque fraîche*: big fruit with very juicy red flesh.

Fried egg★★★/*Œuf au plat*: lightly cooked egg, not scrambled, in an oiled frying pan.
Note: cook it without fat.

Fried food/*Friture*: cf. "Fry".

Frikandel★★★/*Fricadelle*: small ball of ground meat.

Fritter/*Beignet*: fried dish consisting of a piece of meat, fruit, vegetable, etc. wrapped in a thick batter or breading.

Frog's leg★★★/*Cuisse de grenouille*: edible frog's leg.
Note: cook it without fat: en papillote, in water, grill...

Fromage à la pie★★/*Fromage à la pie*: cow's milk fromage frais with herbs. Dairy product.
Note: do not consume more than approximately ½ oz of cheese three times per week... and never at dinner.

Fructose★★/*Fructose*: component of the sugar used as sweetener.

Fruit bar/*Barre de fruits*: very sugary bar made of various dried or fresh fruits.

Fruit compote★★★/*Compote de fruit*: mix of fresh or dried fruits cooked with a little bit of water and added sugar.

Fruit compote with no added sugar ★★★/*Compote de fruit sans sucre ajouté*: mix of fresh or dried fruits cooked without added sugar.

Fruit in light syrup/*Fruit au sirop léger*: fruit poached in a syrup made of water and a small quantity of sugar.

Fruit in light syrup cocktail/*Cocktail de fruit au sirop léger*: mix of various fruits cut in dices and poached before being preserved in more or less sugary water.

Fruit in syrup/*Fruit au sirop*: poached fruit preserved in a syrup made of water and sugar.

Fruit in syrup cocktail/*Cocktail de fruit au sirop*: mix of various fruits cut in dices and poached before being preserved in very sugary water.

Fruit jelly(1)/*Gelée de fruit*: fruit juice cooked with sugar and which hardens when cooling.

Fruit jelly(2)/*Pâte de fruit*: confection made of fruit purée and sugar.

Fruit juice with pulp★/*Jus de fruit avec pulpe*: 100% pure juice fruit juice with the pulp.

Fruit Melba/*Fruit Melba*: fruit poached in syrup before being served on a layer of vanilla ice cream and coated with whipped cream.

Fruit nectar/*Nectar de fruits*: beverage made of fruit purée with water and sugar.

Fruit pectin/*Pectine de fruit*: very sugary substance extracted from fruits used to set jams and sugar-coat pastries.

Fruit salad in light syrup/*Salade de fruits au sirop léger*: mix of various fresh fruits preserved in their low-sugar poaching syrup.

Fruit salad in syrup/*Salade de fruits au sirop*: mix of various poached fruits preserved in their poaching syrup.

Fruit specialty/*Spécialité de fruit*: fruit cooked with fructose and fruit pectin.

Fruit yogurt★★★/*Yaourt aux fruits*: cow's milk, goat milk or sheep milk fermented thanks to lactic acid bacteria and in which fruits have been added. Dairy product.
Note: do not consume if it's sweetened.

Fucus vesiculosus★★★/*Fucus vésiculeux*: edible seaweed.

Fufu★★★/*Foufou*: cassava flour cooked in water and served under the shape of a ball. Gluten-free.

G

Galantine★/*Galantine*: cooked meat made of lean meat and stuffing covered with jelly.

Galette bretonne/*Galette bretonne*: plain cookie rich in sugar and butter.

Galloway cheese★: raw or pasteurised cow's milk cheese. Dairy product.
Note: do not consume more than approximately ½ oz of cheese three times per week... and never at dinner.

Game★★★/*Gibier*: all wild animals hunted for their meat.
Note: do not consume more than approximately 4 oz of red meat twice per week. Cook it without fat: en papillote, in water, grill, roast...

Ganache★/*Crème ganache*: chocolate custard with butter and crème fraîche.
Note: do not consume if it's sweetened.

Gaperon★/*Gaperon*: soft raw cow's milk cheese flavored with garlic. Dairy product.
Note: do not consume more than approximately ½ oz of cheese three times per week... and never at dinner.

Garden orache: cf. "Atriplex hortensis".

Garden sage★★★/*Thé d'Europe*: infusion of heath speedwell leaves.
Note: do not consume if it's sweetened.

Garfish★★★/*Orphie*: long, thin and fatty saltwater fish.
Note: cook it without fat: en papillote, grill, roast...

Garlic★★★/*Ail*: vegetable bulb-plant which cloves are used when cooking. Green vegetable.

Garlic pulp/Pulpe d'ail: cf. "Garlic".

Garlic salt★★★/*Sel d'ail*: mix of table salt and dehydrated garlic in powder.

Garlic sausage/*Saucisson à l'ail*: big sausage eaten cooked. Cooked meat.

Garlic semolina★★★/*Ail semoule*: dehydrated and crushed garlic.

Gazpacho★★★/*Gaspacho*: soup made of raw vegetables macerated in cold water and served very fresh. Green vegetable.

Gelatin★★★/*Gélatine*: collagen sheet which dissolves in hot water to make jellies.

Genoise/*Génoise*: light cookie dough used as the base of numerous cakes.

Germinated adzuki bean seed★★★/*Graine de haricot azuki germée*: adzuki bean seed eaten germinated.

**Germinated barley seed
- Germinated wheat seed**

Germinated barley seed★★★/*Graine d'orge germée*: barley seed eaten germinated.

Germinated buckwheat seed★★★/*Graine de sarrasin germée*: buckwheat seed eaten germinated.

Germinated chickpea seed★★★/*Graine de pois chiche germée*: chickpea seed eaten germinated.

Germinated corn grain★★★/*Graine de maïs germée*: corn grain eaten germinated.

Germinated lentil seed★★★/*Graine de lentille germée*: lentil seed eaten germinated.

Germinated millet seed★★★/*Graine de millet germée*: millet seed eaten germinated.

Germinated mung bean seed★★★/*Graine de haricot mungo germée*: muni bean seed eaten germinated.

Germinated oats seed★★★/*Graine d'avoine germée*: oats seed eaten germinated.

Germinated pea seed★★★/*Graine de petit pois germée*: pea seed eaten germinated.

Germinated rice seed★★★/*Graine de riz germée*: rice seed eaten germinated.

Germinated rye seed★★★/*Graine de seigle germée*: rye seed eaten germinated.

Germinated spelt seed★★★/*Graine d'épeautre germée*: spelt seed eaten germinated.

Germinated wheat seed★★★/*Graine de blé germée*: wheat seed eaten germinated.

Giblets★★★/Abats de volaille: edible offal of a fowl, typically including the heart, gizzard, liver, and other organs.
Note: cook it without fat or with olive oil.

Gigot★★/Gigot: lamb, sheep or deer posterior. Red meat.
Note: do not consume more than approximately 4 oz of red meat twice per week. Cook it without fat: en papillote, in water, grill, roast...

Gin/Gin: grain eau de vie flavored with juniper berries.

Ginger★★★/Gingembre: aromatic rhizome used as a condiment. Green vegetable.

Gingerbread/Pain d'épice: cake made of rye flour with sugar, honey and seasoning. Carbohydrate.

Gizzard★★★/Gésier: poultry stomach. Offal.
Note: cook it without fat or with olive oil.

Glucose/Glucose: carbohydrate, quick sugar.

Gluten★★★/Gluten: protein part of the following cereals: wheat, rye, barley and oats.

Gluten-free bagel★★/Bagel sans gluten: small white bread shaped into a ring with very firm gluten-free crumb. Carbohydrate.

Gluten-free beer★/Bière sans gluten: drink from the alcoholic fermentation of mainly barley and from which the gluten is extracted.
Note: do not drink alcoholic beverage, however no problem if it's cooked.

Gluten-free bread★★★/Pain sans gluten: bread made of gluten-free flour. Carbohydrate.

Gluten-free breadcrumbs★★★/*Chapelure sans gluten*: gluten-free white bread toasted in the oven before being crushed into crumbs. Carbohydrate.

Gluten-free breakfast sugary extruded cereal/*Céréale extrudée sucrée pour petit-déjeuner sans gluten*: gluten-free swelled cereal coated in sugar, honey, chocolat, etc. Carbohydrate.

Gluten-free bun★★★/*Bun sans gluten*: small round and puffy gluten-free bread. Carbohydrate.

Gluten-free cake(1)/*Cake sans gluten*: cake made of gluten-free egg batter with yeast, candied fruits and raisins soaked in rum.

Gluten-free cake(2)/*Gâteau sans gluten*: pastry made of a gluten-free batter used alone or with a cream, fruits...

Gluten-free cannellonis★★★/*Cannelloni sans gluten*: gluten-free pasta rolled in the shape of a cylinder and stuffed with stuffing. Carbohydrate.

Gluten-free cookie/*Biscuit sans gluten*: cookie that does not contain gluten. Carbohydrate.

Gluten-free crepe★★★/*Crêpe sans gluten*: crepe made of gluten-free flour.
Note: do not consume if it's sweetened.

Gluten-free crispbread★★/*Biscotte sans gluten*: slice of gluten-free sandwich bread industrially toasted in the oven. Carbohydrate.

Gluten-free crouton★★★/*Croûton sans gluten*: small piece of fried gluten-free white bread. Carbohydrate.

Gluten-free kringle★★/*Craquelin sans gluten*: small crispy cookie made of an unleavened and gluten-free batter.

Gluten-free madeleine/*Madeleine sans gluten*: small cake in the shape of a bulging shell made of gluten-free flour.

Gluten-free margarine★★/*Margarine sans gluten*: gluten-free plant-based dietary fats.
Note: consume it in moderation. Do not cook with it.

Gluten-free muffin★★★/*Muffin sans gluten*: small plain bread with leaven but without gluten. Carbohydrate.

Gluten-free pancakes★★★/*Pancakes sans gluten*: small thick crepe made of gluten-free sieved flour. Carbohydrate.
Note: do not consume if it's sweetened.

Gluten-free pie crust★★★/*Pâte brisée sans gluten*: crust made of gluten-free flour, butter and eggs. Carbohydrate.

Gluten-free pizza base★★★/*Pâte à pizza sans gluten*: base made of gluten-free flour, water and yeast.

Gluten-free pretzel/*Bretzel sans gluten*: gluten-free cookie into an 8-shape, sprinkled with salt and cumin.

Gluten-free puff pastry★★★/*Pâte feuilletée sans gluten*: pastry made of gluten-free flour, butter and eggs. Carbohydrate.

Gluten-free sweet shortcrust pastry/*Pâte sablée sans gluten*: pastry made of gluten-free flour, sugar, butter and eggs.

Gluten-free toast★★★/*Toast sans gluten*: slice of gluten-free toasted bread.

Gluten-free whole-grain cannellonis ★★★/*Cannelloni complet sans gluten*: whole-grain gluten-free pasta rolled in the shape of a cylinder and stuffed with stuffing. Carbohydrate.

**Gluten-free whole-grain muffin
- Goat milk cottage cheese**

Gluten-free whole-grain muffin★★★/*Muffin complet sans gluten*: small plain whole-grain bread with leaven but without gluten. Carbohydrate.

Gluten-free wholewheat breadcrumbs ★★★/*Chapelure complète sans gluten*: gluten-free wholewheat bread toasted in the oven before being crushed into crumbs. Carbohydrate.

Gluten-free wholewheat crepe★★★/*Crêpe complète sans gluten*: thin layer of cooked batter made of eggs, milk and gluten-free wholewheat flour. Carbohydrate.
Note: do not consume if it's sweetened.

Gluten-free wholewheat crouton★★★/*Croûton complet sans gluten*: small piece of fried gluten-free wholewheat bread. Carbohydrate.

Gluten-free wholewheat pancakes★★★/*Pancakes complet sans gluten*: small thick crepes made of gluten-free wholewheat flour. Carbohydrate.
Note: do not consume if it's sweetened.

Gluten-free wholewheat toast★★★/*Toast complet sans gluten*: slice of gluten-free wholewheat toasted bread.

Gnocchi★★★/*Gnocchi*: ball made of wheat semolina and potatoes. Carbohydrate.

Goat milk cheese★/*Fromage de chèvre*: cheese made of goat milk. Dairy product.
Note: do not consume more than approximately ½ oz of cheese three times per week... and never at dinner.

Goat milk cottage cheese★★★/*Faisselle au lait de chèvre*: fresh cheese made of goat milk. Dairy product.
Note: the less fat, the better!

Goat milk cream dessert/*Crème dessert au lait de chèvre*: dairy specialty or dessert made of goat milk, sugar and eggs. Dairy product.

Goat milk fromage blanc★★★/*Fromage blanc de chèvre*: fresh cheese made of goat milk, a bit drained and not aged. Dairy product.
Note: the less fat, the better!

Goat's cheese log★/*Bûche de chèvre*: goat milk cheese in the shape of a small round and long cylinder. Dairy product.
Note: do not consume more than approximately ½ oz of cheese three times per week... and never at dinner.

Good-king-Henry: cf. "Blitum bonus-henricus".

Goose★★★/*Oie*: massive palmiped bird. Poultry.
Note: cook it without fat: en papillote, in water, grill, roast...

Goose fat/*Graisse d'oie*: goose fat used to make confits.

Goose rillettes/*Rillettes d'oie*: cooked meat made of goose meat cooked in its fat.

Gorgonzola★/*Gorgonzola*: cow's milk cheese with parsley in it. Dairy product.
Note: do not consume more than approximately ½ oz of cheese three times per week... and never at dinner.

Gouda★/*Gouda*: pressed and raw cow's milk cheese. Dairy product.
Note: do not consume more than approximately ½ oz of cheese three times per week... and never at dinner.

Gougère★/*Gougère*: salted choux pastry with gruyère baked in the oven.
Note: do not consume more than approximately ½ oz of cheese three times per week... and never at dinner.

Goulash - Green laver

Goulash★★★/*Goulache*: stew made of simmered meat, onions, tomatoes and paprika.

Grapefruit in light syrup/*Pamplemousse au sirop léger*: poached grapefruit preserved in more or less sugary water.

Grapefruit in syrup/*Pamplemousse au sirop*: poached grapefruit preserved in very sugary water.

Grapefruit juice★/*Jus de pamplemousse*: juice made of the pressing of grapefruits.

Grape juice★/*Jus de raisin*: juice made of the pressing of grapes.

Grape seed oil★★/*Huile de pépin de raisin*: fatty substance made of grape seeds.

Grated coconut/*Noix de coco râpée*: cf. "Coconut". Exotic fruit.

Gratin★★/*Gratin*: dish covered with breadcrumbs or cheese baked in the oven.
Note: do not consume more than approximately ½ oz of cheese three times per week... and never at dinner.

Grayling★★★/*Ombre*: fatty freshwater fish.
Note: cook it without fat: en papillote, in water, grill, roast...

Grecque (à la)★★★/*Grecque (à la)*: cooked in an olive oil and seasoning marinade, eaten cold.

Greek yogurt/*Yaourt à la grecque*: cf. "Yogurt".

Green bean★★★/*Haricot vert*: green or violet bean, sometimes green with black stripes or brown, chocolate... eaten young. Green vegetable.

Green laver★★★/*Ao-nori*: edible green seaweeds.

Green tea★★★/*Thé vert*: infusion of tea bush leaves roasted after being picked.
Note: do not consume if it's sweetened.

Green vegetable cream soup/*Velouté de légumes verts*: cf. "Green vegetable soup".

Green vegetable/*Légume vert*: vegetable plant from which, depending on the variety, we eat the leaves, the chards, the stems, the roots or the fruits. See each green vegetable separately.

Green vegetable soup★★★/*Potage de légumes verts*: mixed vegetable stock.

Green vegetable soup in carton★★★/*Potage de légumes verts en brique*: industrial soup ready to be drunk.

Grenadine/*Grenadine*: syrup flavored with red berry juice and vanilla.

Grenadine juice★/*Jus de grenade*: juice made of the pressing of pomegranates. Exotic fruit.

Grilled buckwheat★★★/*Sarrasin grillé*: grilled buckwheat seed ready to be eaten.

Grilled food★★★/*Grillade*: slice of meat or grilled fish.

Grilletine/*Grilletine*: slice of brioche toasted in the oven. Carbohydrate.

Grissino★★/*Gressin*: small white bread made with an egg batter. Carbohydrate.

Ground beef steak with vegetable protein★★/*Steak haché de bœuf avec protéines végétales*: ground beef steak containing 80% of ground beef meat and 20% of vegetable proteins.

Ground (food)★★★/*Haché (aliment)*: food that is ground before being eaten.

Ground ham steak★★★/*Steak haché de jambon*: ground pork meat.
Note: cook it without fat: grill, roast...

Ground meat★★★/*Hachis*: dish made of ground meat, fish, green vegetables.

Groundnut★/*Arachide*: envelope of the peanut.

Groundnut butter/*Beurre d'arachide*: cf. "Peanut".

Ground veal steak★★★/*Steak haché de veau*: ground veal meat.
Note: cook it without fat: grill, roast...

Grouper★★★/*Mérou*: saltwater fish with white flesh found in hot waters.
Note: cook it without fat: en papillote, in water, grill, roast...

Gruel★★/*Gruau*: hard wheat semolina. Carbohydrate.

Gruel flour★★★/*Farine de gruau*: sieved and very thin wheat of high quality flour. Carbohydrate.

Gruyère★/*Gruyère*: hard cow's milk with washed rind. Dairy product.
Note: do not consume more than approximately ½ oz of cheese three times per week... and never at dinner.

Guacamole★/*Guacamole*: dish made of avocados, tomatoes, onions, crème fraîche and spices.

Guar gum★★★/*Gomme de guar*: vegetable thickening substance.

Guava in light syrup/*Goyave au sirop léger*: poached guava preserved in more or less sugary water. Exotic fruit.

Guava in syrup/*Goyave au sirop*: poached guava preserved in very sugary water. Exotic fruit.

Guava jelly/*Pâte de goyave*: sugary guava marmalade.

Guava juice/*Jus de goyave*: juice made of the pressing of guavas. Exotic fruit.

Gudgeon★★★/*Goujon*: small freshwater fish with white flesh.
Note: cook it without fat.

Guinea fowl★★★/*Pintade*: bird a little bit smaller than chicken.
Note: cook it without fat: en papillote, in water, grill, roast...

Gurnard★★★/*Grondin*: saltwater fish with white flesh.
Note: cook it without fat: en papillote, in water, grill, roast...

H

Haddock★★★/*Eglefin*: saltwater fish with white flesh.
Note: cook it without fat: en papillote, in water, grill, roast...

Halbi/*Halbi*: beverage made of a mix of fermented apples and pears.

Halibut★★★/*Flétan*: big saltwater fish with white flesh.
Note: cook it without fat: en papillote, in water, grill, roast...

Halibut liver oil★★/*Huile de foie de flétan*: fatty substance made of halibut liver.

Halva/*Halva*: confection made of flour, sesame oil, dried fruits and honey.

Ham★★★/*Jambon blanc*: cooked and boneless pork ham. Cooked meat.
Note: cook it without fat.

Ham allumette★★★/*Allumette de jambon*: matchstick-sized cut of ham.
Note: cook it without fat.

Ham and cheese escalope★★/*Cordon bleu de jambon*: pork escalope wrapped around ham and cheese.
Note: cook it without fat.

Hamburger(1)★★/*Hamburger(1)*: ground steak in a small round bun. Red meat.
Note: do not consume more than approximately 4 oz of red meat twice per week. Cook it without fat.

Hamburger(2)★★/*Hamburger(2)*: ground steak with a fried egg. Red meat.
Note: do not consume more than approximately 4 oz of red meat twice per week. Cook it without fat. Do not consume more than 3 eggs per week.

Ham ravioli★★★/*Ravioli au jambon*: small square of pasta stuffed with pork meat, ground herbs, etc. before being poached. Carbohydrate.

Hang★★★/*Faisander*: to give a strong fumet to game letting it start rotting.

Hanger steak★★/*Onglet*: piece of beef from which we cut tasty beefsteaks. Red meat.
Note: do not consume more than approximately 4 oz of red meat twice per week. Cook it without fat: en papillote, in water, grill, roast...

Hard-boiled egg★★★/*Œuf dur*: egg cooked in a lot of water.

Hare★★★/_Lièvre_: kind of wild rabbit. Game.
Note: cook it without fat: en papillote, in water, grill, roast...

Harissa★★★/_Harissa_: condiment made of chili pepper and oil.

Haunch★★/_Cuissot_: wild boar's leg, venison's leg or deer's leg. Red meat. Game.
Note: do not consume more than approximately 4 oz of red meat twice per week. Cook it without fat: en papillote, in water, grill, roast...

Hazelnut★★/_Noisette_: nut from the hazel.

Hazelnut cream★★★/_Crème de noisette_: more or less liquid cream made of hazelnut milk, substitute to crème fraîche.

Hazelnut milk★★★/_Lait de noisette_: plant milk from hazelnuts. Lactose-free.
Note: do not consume if it's sweetened.

Hazelnut milk cream dessert/_Crème dessert au lait de noisette_: vegetable dessert made of hazelnut milk, sugar and eggs. Dairy product.

Hazelnut milk yogurt★★★/_Yaourt au lait de noisette_: hazelnut milk fermented thanks to lactic acid bacteria, sweetened or not. Dairy product. Lactose-free.
Note: do not consume if it's sweetened.

Hazelnut oil★★/_Huile de noisette_: fatty substance made of hazelnut.

Hazelnut purée★★/_Purée de noisette_: mashed hazelnuts to spread.

Hazelnut spread/_Pâte à tartiner de noisette_: very sugary and fat mix of crushed hazelnuts.

Head cheese★/*Fromage de tête*: cooked meat. Pâté made of pork head pieces with jelly.

Headcheese★/*Museau*: cooked meat dish made of pork or beef chin and nose.

Heart★★★/*Cœur*: butcher's meat. Offal.
Note: cook it without fat: to grill, to roast, etc.

Heavy crème fraîche/*Crème fraîche entière*: fats from unsterilized milk (30%) with which the butter is made. Made of raw milk. Dairy product.

Heifer lamb★★/*Rognon de génisse*: kidney of the heifer. Offal.
Note: cook it without fat: to grill, to roast, etc.

Heifer liver★★/*Foie de génisse*: offal.
Note: cook it without fat: to grill, to roast, etc.

Helianthus strumosus★★★/*Hélianti*: vegetable plant from which we eat the rhizome. Green vegetable.

Helvella★★★/*Helvelle*: edible wild mushroom. Green vegetable.

Hemp cream★★★/*Crème de chanvre*: more or less liquid cream made of hemp milk, substitute to crème fraîche.

Hemp milk★★★/*Lait de chanvre*: plant milk from hemps. Lactose-free.
Note: do not consume if it's sweetened.

Hemp milk cream dessert/*Crème dessert au lait de chanvre*: vegetable dessert made of hemp milk, sugar and eggs. Dairy product.

Hemp oil★★/*Huile de chanvre*: fatty substance made of hemp.

Hemp seed★★★/*Graine de chanvre*: hemp seed eaten crushed or germinated.

Hen★★★/*Poule*: female rooster. Needs to be cooked for a long time, in sauce or boiled. Poultry.
Note: cook it without fat: en papillote, in water...

Herbal tea★★★/*Infusion*: liquid in which a plant is put to infuse.
Note: do not consume if it's sweetened.

Herbs★★★/*Herbes (fines)*: aromatic and edible plants used as condiments: parsley, dill, chive, etc.

Herring★★★/*Hareng*: fatty saltwater fish.
Note: cook it without fat: en papillote, in water, grill, roast...

Hijiki★★★/*Hijiki*: edible black seaweed.

Himanthalia elongata★★★/*Haricot de mer*: edible seaweed.

Hog/*Cochon*: cf. "Pork (meat)".

Hollandaise sauce★/*Sauce hollandaise*: sauce made of egg yolks and butter.

Honey/*Miel*: very sugary substance produced by bees.

Hoop cheese★: pasteurised cow's milk cheese. Dairy product.
Note: do not consume more than approximately ½ oz of cheese three times per week... and never at dinner.

Horse (meat)★★★/*Cheval (viande de...)*: red meat, butcher meat.
Cook it without fat: en papillote, in water, grill, roast...

Horseradish★★★/*Raifort*: vegetable plant grown for its plump and pepper flavored root. Green vegetable.

**Horseradish seed
- Iced chocolate with whipped cream**

Horseradish seed★★★/*Graine de raifort*: horseradish seed eaten crushed or germinated.

Horse spider steak★★★/*Araignée de cheval*: piece of very tender meat from the horse's pelvis muscles. Red meat.

Host★★★/*Hostie*: eucharistic bread made of leaven-free flour. Carbohydrate.

Hot dog★★/*Hot dog*: small hot bread with a sausage and mustard.

Hot pot★★/*Fondue chinoise*: dish made of small dices of beef dipped in meat or poultry stock.
Note: do not consume more than approximately 4 oz of red meat twice per week.

Humboldt fog cheese★: pasteurised goat's milk cheese. Dairy product.
Note: do not consume more than approximately ½ oz of cheese three times per week... and never at dinner.

Hummus/*Houmous*★★★: mix of tahini and mashed split peas. Carbohydrate.

I

Ice cream(1)/*Crème glacée*: dessert made of cream, milk, sugar and flavors with sometimes egg yolks.

Ice cream(2)/*Glace*: frozen cream made of milk, sugar, eggs fruit-flavored or fruits with fruits.

Iced chocolate with whipped cream/*Liégeois (chocolat)*: chocolate ice cream coated with whipped cream.

Iced tea/*Thé glacé*: infusion of sugary tea drunk fresh.

Industrial ready-cooked dishes★★/*Plat cuisiné industriel*: various dishes sold vacuum packed, frozen or fresh, industrially made and ready to be eaten.
Note: do not consume if it's sweetened.

Industrial sandwich bread★★/*Pain de mie industriel*: crustless bread made of white flour, industrially produced and sold pre-sliced. Carbohydrate.

Industrial tomato sauce★★★/*Sauce tomate cuisinée*: industrially cooked tomatoes with flavors, meat, additives, etc. found in cans.

Industrial vinaigrette sauce★★★/*Sauce vinaigrette industrielle*: sauce industrially made of vegetable oil and vinegar.

Industrial wholewheat sandwich bread★★★/*Pain de mie complet industriel*: crustless bread made of wholewheat or semi wholewheat flour, industrially produced and sold pre-sliced. Carbohydrate.

Infant formula milk★★★/*Lait pour nourrisson*: food preparation made to replace human breast milk if the mother cannot or do not want to breastfeed her baby.
Note: do not consume if it's sweetened.

Irish coffee/*Irish-coffee*: coffee with Irish whiskey and coated with crème fraîche.

Irish moss★★★/*Mousse d'Irlande*: edible red seaweed.

J

Jackfruit★★★/*Jaque*: fruit from the jackfruit tree eaten raw as a vegetable.

Jam/*Confiture*: mix of fresh fruits and sugar cooked together.

Jam with no sugar★★/*Confiture sans sucre*: mix of fruits and sweetener(s) and/or fruit sugar.

John dory★★★/*Saint-pierre*: saltwater fish with white flesh.
Note: cook it without fat: en papillote, in water, grill, roast...

Jonchée cheese★/*Jonchée*: cow's milk, sheep milk or goat milk cheese in a bulrush basket. Dairy product.
Note: do not consume more than approximately ½ oz of cheese three times per week... and never at dinner.

Jujube in light syrup/*Jujube au sirop léger*: poached jujube preserved in more or less sugary water. Exotic fruit.

Jujube in syrup/*Jujube au sirop*: poached jujube preserved in very sugary water. Exotic fruit.

Jumbo shrimp★★★/*Langoustine*: crustacean the size of a big crawfish.
Note: cook it without fat: en papillote, in water, grill, roast...

Junk-food/Fast-food: fast food.

K

Kaki in light syrup/*Kaki au sirop léger*: poached kaki preserved in more or less sugary water.

Kaki in syrup/*Kaki au sirop*: poached kaki preserved in very sugary water.

Kale★★★/*Chou frisé*: vegetable plant from which we eat all the leaves.

Kangaroo (meat of...)★★/*Kangourou (viande de...)*: meat similar to that of beef. Red meat.
Note: do not consume more than approximately 4 oz of red meat twice per week. Cook it without fat: en papillote, in water, grill, roast...

Kefir★★/*Kéfir*: fizzy fermented beverage made of cow's milk, goat milk, sheep milk or she-camel milk. Dairy product.

Ketchup/*Ketchup*: thick spicy sauce made of tomatoes and sugar.

Khorasan wheat flake★★★/*Flocon de kamut*: small portion of dehydrated khorasan wheat. Carbohydrate.

Khorasan wheat flour★★★/*Farine de kamut*: powder made of refined khorasan wheat milling. Carbohydrate.

Khorasan wheat milk★★★/*Lait de kamut*: plant milk from Khorasan wheat. Lactose-free.
Note: do not consume if it's sweetened.

Khorasan wheat pasta★★★/*Pâte alimentaire de kamut*: mix to be cooked made of refined khorasan wheat. Carbohydrate.

Kidney bean★★★/*Haricot rouge*: red bean seed eaten fully ripe. Carbohydrate.

Kig ha far★★/*Kig ha far*: pork stew in which a mix of wheat or buckwheat is cooked. Carbohydrate.

King shrimp★★★/*Gamba*: very big shrimp.
Note: cook it without fat: en papillote, in water, grill...

Kipper★★★/*Kipper*: herring which head has been removed before opening the fish and smoking it.
Note: cook it without fat: en papillote, grill, roast...

Kir royal/*Kir royal*: champagne with blackcurrant liqueur.

Kir/*Kir*: white wine with blackcurrant liqueur.

Kirsch★/*Kirsch*: cherry eau de vie.
Note: do not drink alcoholic beverage, however no problem if it's cooked.

Kiwi in light syrup/*Kiwi au sirop léger*: poached kiwi preserved in more or less sugary water.

Kiwi in syrup/*Kiwi au sirop*: poached kiwi preserved in very sugary water.

Kiwi juice★/*Jus de kiwi*: juice made of the pressing of kiwis.

Kohlrabi★★★/*Chou-rave*: vegetable plant from which we eat the stem bulge.

Kombu★★★/*Kombu*: edible seaweed.

Kringle★★/*Craquelin*: small crispy cookie made of an unleavened batter.
Note: do not consume if it's sweetened.

Kumis★/Koumis: fermented beverage made of cow's milk, mare's milk or she-camel milk. Dairy product.

Kumquat in light syrup/*Kumquat au sirop léger*: poached kumquat preserved in more or less sugary water.

Kumquat in syrup/*Kumquat au sirop*: poached kumquat preserved in very sugary water.

Kvass/*Kwas*: alcoholic beverage made of fermented barley or rye flour.

L

Lactose-free butter★★/*Beurre sans lactose*: unsalted dietary fats made from the cream of lactose-free cow's milk.
Note: consume it in moderation. Do not cook with it. The less fat, the better!

Lactose-free fromage blanc★★★/*Fromage blanc sans lactose*: fresh cheese made of lactose-free milk, a bit drained and not aged. Dairy product.
Note: the less fat, the better!

Lactose-free margarine★★/*Margarine sans lactose*: lactose-free plant-based dietary fats.
Note: consume it in moderation. Do not cook with it.

Lactose-free petit suisse★★★/*Petit-suisse sans lactose*: plain petit suisse made of lactose-free milk.
Note: the less fat, the better!

Lactose-free semi-skimmed milk★★/*Lait demi-écrémé délactosé*: lactose-free mammal milk which has been semi skimmed.

Lactose-free skimmed milk★★★/*Lait écrémé délactosé*: skimmed mammal milk without lactose.

Lactose-free whole milk/*Lait entier délactosé*: whole mammal milk without lactose.

Lactose-free yogurt★★★/*Yaourt sans lactose*: mammal milk yogurt without lactose. Dairy product.
Note: the less fat, the better!

Ladyfinger/*Boudoir*: long cookie sprinkled with sugar.

Laguiole cheese★/*Laguiole*: raw cow's milk cheese close to Cantal cheese. Dairy product.
Note: do not consume more than approximately ½ oz of cheese three times per week... and never at dinner.

Lamb breast★★/*Poitrine d'agneau*: inferior part of the lamb's rib cage to boil or to simmer. Red meat.
Note: do not consume more than approximately 4 oz of red meat twice per week. Cook it without fat: en papillote, in water, grill, roast...

Lamb kidney★★/*Rognon d'agneau*: kidney of the lamb. Offal.
Note: cook it without fat: grill, roast...

Lamb liver★★★/*Foie d'agneau*: offal.
Note: cook it without fat: en papillote, grill, roast...

Lamb (meat)/*Agneau (viande d')*: baby of the sheep. Red meat. See each piece separately.

Lamb neck★★/*Collet d'agneau*: piece of lamb meat to boil or to simmer. Red meat.
Note: do not consume more than approximately 4 oz of red meat twice per week. Cook it without fat: en papillote, in water, grill, roast...

Lamb rib★★/*Côte d'agneau*: anterior part of the lamb. Red meat.
Note: do not consume more than approximately 4 oz of red meat twice per week. Cook it without fat: en papillote, in water, grill, roast...

Lamb shoulder★★/*Palette d'agneau*: lamb shoulder blade and the flesh around it. Red meat.
Note: do not consume more than approximately 4 oz of red meat twice per week. Cook it without fat: en papillote, in water, grill, roast...

Lamb's lettuce★★★/*Mâche*: vegetable plant from which we eat the leaves in salad. Green vegetable.

Lamb stew with beans★★/*Haricot de mouton*: lamb stew with dried beans or java beans.
Note: do not consume more than approximately 4 oz of red meat twice per week. Cook it without fat: en papillote, in water, grill, roast...

Lamb sweetbread★★/*Ris d'agneau*: lamb thymus. Offal.
Note: cook it without fat or with olive oil.

Lamprey★★★/*Lamproie*: fish with white flesh found in rivers.
Note: cook it without fat: en papillote, in water, grill, roast...

Lanark blue★: raw or pasteurised sheep's milk cheese. Dairy product.
Note: do not consume more than approximately ½ oz of cheese three times per week... and never at dinner.

Lancashire cheese★: pasteurised cow's milk cheese. Dairy product.
Note: do not consume more than approximately ½ oz of cheese three times per week... and never at dinner.

Langres cheese★/*Langres*: soft and fermented cow's milk cheese.
Note: do not consume more than approximately ½ oz of cheese three times per week... and never at dinner.

Langue de chat biscuit/*Langue-de-chat*: small plain cookie in the shape of a rounded tongue.

Lapsang souchong★★★/*Souchong*: Chinese black tea.
Note: do not consume if it's sweetened.

Lard(1)/*Larder*: prick a meat with small pieces of bacon.

Lard(2)/*Saindoux*: pork fat.

Larded (meat)★/*Entrelardée (viande)*: slice of meat relatively fat.
Note: cook it without fat: to grill, to roast, etc.

Largemouth bass★★★/*Black-Bass*: fatty freshwater fish.
Note: cook it without fat: en papillote, in water, grill, roast...

Lasagna★★★/*Lasagne(1)*: dish made of pasta, tomato sauce, ground beef meat and bechamel sauce baked in the oven. Carbohydrate.
Note: do not consume more than approximately 4 oz of red meat twice per week.

Lasagna sheet★★★/*Lasagne(2)*: pasta in the shape of large flat patches. Carbohydrate.

Lathyrus sativus★★★/*Gesse commune*: vegetable plant from which we eat the cooked seeds. Green vegetable.

Leaf cabbage/*Chou kale*: cf. "Kale".

Lean fish★★★/*Poisson maigre*: fish with white flesh, moderately rich in polyunsaturated fats and in omega 3: sole, cod, pollock, gurnard, carp, roach, pike, zander, etc.
Note: cook it without fat: en papillote, in water, grill, roast...

Lean fish fillet★★★/*Filet de poisson maigre*: slice of fish with white flesh in general without fishbone.
Note: cook it without fat: en papillote, in water, grill, roast...

Lean (meat or fish)★★★/*Maigre (viande ou poisson)*: meat or fish containing very low quantities of fat.
Note: cook it without fat: to grill, to roast, etc.

Leaven★★★/*Levain*: piece of batter being fermented mixed to bread batter to make it rise and ferment it.

Leek★★★/*Poireau*: vegetable plant entirely edible. Green vegetable.

Leek seed★★★/*Graine de poireau*: leek seed eaten crushed or germinated.

Leg of deer★★/*Gigue*: deer leg. Game. Red meat.
Note: do not consume more than approximately 4 oz of red meat twice per week. Cook it without fat: en papillote, in water, grill, roast...

Lemon balm★★★/*Mélisse*: aromatic plant used as a condiment.

Lemon curd/*Crème de citron*: spread made of butter, sugar and lemon.

Lemon in light syrup/*Citron au sirop léger*: poached lemon preserved in more or less sugary water.

Lemon in syrup/*Citron au sirop*: poached lemon preserved in sugary water.

Lemon juice★★★/*Jus de citron*: juice made of the pressing of lemons.

Lemonade/*Citronnade*: beverage made of lemon juice and sugary water.

Lemongrass★★★/*Citronnelle*: grass used as an aromatic plant.

Lemon soda/*Limonade*: fizzy beverage made of sugar, lemon essence and carbon dioxide.

Lentil★★★/*Lentille*: annual plant grown for its seeds which are dried legumes. Carbohydrate.

Lentil flake★★★/*Flocon de lentille*: small portion of dehydrated lentil. Carbohydrate. Gluten-free.

Lentil flour★★★/*Farine de lentille*: powder made of lentil milling. Gluten-free.

Lentil pasta★★★/*Pâte alimentaire de lentille*: mix to be cooked made of lentil flour. Carbohydrate. Gluten-free.

Lesser sand eel★★★/*Equille*: small and elongated saltwater fish with white flesh.
Note: cook it without fat: en papillote, in water...

Lettuce★★★/*Laitue*: annual vegetable plant eaten in salad. Green vegetable.

Licorice/*Réglisse*: small confection aniseed-flavored.

Liederkranz cheese★: cow's milk cheese with pasteurized milk. Dairy product.
Note: do not consume more than approximately ½ oz of cheese three times per week... and never at dinner.

Light fruit compote★★★/*Compote de fruit allégée*: mix of fresh or dried fruits cooked with a little bit of water and added sugar.

Light iced tea★★★/*Thé glacé light*: infusion of sweetened tea in bottle drunk fresh, sugar-free.

Light industrial ready-cooked dishes★★★/*Plat cuisiné industriel light*: various low-fat dishes sold vacuum packed, frozen or fresh, industrially made and ready to be eaten.
Note: do not consume if it's sweetened.

Light industrial vinaigrette sauce★★★/*Sauce vinaigrette industrielle allégée*: sauce industrially made of vegetable oil and vinegar and containing low quantities of fats.

Lightly salted butter★★/*Beurre demi-sel allégé*: salted dietary fats made from the cream of cow's milk.
Note: consume it in moderation. Do not cook with it. The less fat, the better!

Lightly salted margarine★★/*Margarine demi-sel allégée*: salted plant-based dietary fats.
Note: consume it in moderation. Do not cook with it.

Light mayonnaise★/*Mayonnaise allégée*: cold sauce made of an emulsion of egg yolks, mustard and oil reduced in fats.

Light sirup★★★/*sirop 0% de sucre*: solution made of water and Sweetener (no sugar).

Light soda★★★/*Soda light*: fizzy beverage made of water, gas and one or several sweetener(s).

Lima bean/*Haricot de lima*: cf. "Fava bean".

Lincolnshire poacher★: cow's milk cheese with raw milk. Dairy product.
Note: do not consume more than approximately ½ oz of cheese three times per week... and never at dinner.

Ling★★★/*Lingue*: saltwater fish with white flesh.
Note: cook it without fat: en papillote, in water, grill, roast...

Linseed oil★★/*Huile de lin*: fatty substance made of linseeds.

Liqueur★/*Liqueur*: strong alcoholic beverage.
Note: do not drink alcoholic beverage, however no problem if it's cooked.

Liquid sterilized UHT cream (from 3,2% to 5% fats)★★★/*Crème stérilisée liquide UHT (de 3,2% à 5% de matières grasses)*: fats from the milk (3,2% to 5%) sterilized with which the butter is made. Made of sterilized UHT milk. Dairy product.

Liquid sterilized UHT cream (from 12% to 15% fats)★★/*Crème stérilisée liquide UHT (de 12% à 15% de matières grasses)*: fats from the milk (12% to 15%) sterilized with which the butter is made. Made of sterilized UHT milk. Dairy product.

Little tunny★★★/*Thonine*: fatty saltwater fish.
Note: cook it without fat: en papillote, in water, grill, roast...

Livarot cheese★/*Livarot*: soft cow's milk cheese with washed rind. Dairy product.
Note: do not consume more than approximately ½ oz of cheese three times per week... and never at dinner.

Liver mousse/*Mousse de foie*: cooked meat made of emulsified liver.

Lobster★★★/*Homard*: sea crustacean appreciated for its delicate flesh.
Note: cook it without fat: en papillote, in water, grill, roast...

Loin of veal★★★/*Rouelle de veau*: thick slice of veal leg.
Note: cook it without fat: en papillote, in water, grill, roast...

Lollipop/*Sucette*: candy made of sugar fixed on a stick. Fast-acting sugar.

Longan in light syrup/*Longane au sirop léger*: poached longan preserved in more or less sugary water. Exotic fruit.

Longan in syrup/*Longane au sirop*: poached longan preserved in very sugary water. Exotic fruit.

Lovage★★★/*Livèche*: plant from which we eat the seeds and the fresh leaves. Green vegetable.

Low-fat cow's milk cheese★★/*Fromage de vache allégé en matières grasses*: cheese made of partly skimmed cow's milk. Dairy product.
Note: consume it in moderation. The less fat, the better!

Low-fat fromage blanc★★★/*Fromage blanc allégé en matières grasses*: fresh cheese a bit drained and not aged which contains less fat than usual. Dairy product.
Note: the less fat, the better!

Low-fat goat milk cheese★★/*Fromage de chèvre allégé en matières grasses*: cheese made of partly skimmed goat milk. Dairy product.
Note: consume it in moderation. The less fat, the better!

Low-fat industrial ready-cooked dishes★★★/*Plat cuisiné industriel allégé en matières grasses*: cf. "Light industrial ready-cooked dishes".

Low-fat margarine - Low-sugar breakfast cookie

Low-fat margarine★★/*Margarine allégée en matières grasses*: low-fat plant-based dietary fats.
Note: consume it in moderation. The less fat, the better!

Low-fat petit suisse★★★/*Petit-suisse allégé en matières grasses*: fromage frais in cylindrical shape made of skimmed milk. Dairy product.
Note: consume it in moderation. The less fat, the better!

Low-fat pie crust★★★/*Pâte brisée allégée en matières grasses*: crust made of flour, low-fat butter and eggs. Carbohydrate.

Low-fat puff pastry★★★/*Pâte feuilletée allégée en matières grasses*: pastry made of flour, low-fat butter and eggs. Carbohydrate.

Low-fat sheep cheese★★/*Fromage de brebis allégé en matières grasses*: cheese made of partly skimmed sheep cheese. Dairy product.
Note: consume it in moderation. The less fat, the better!

Low-fat sweet shortcrust pastry/*Pâte sablée allégée en matières grasses*: pastry made of flour, low-fat butter, sugar and eggs. Carbohydrate.

Low-salt food★★★/*Allégé en sel*: a food containing a lower quantity of salt than the original food.

Low-sodium★★★/*Hyposodé*: is said about foods containing low quantities of sodium, so low in salt.

Low-sodium ham★★★/*Jambon blanc à teneur réduite en sel*: boneless pork ham cooked in a low-sodium stock. Cooked meat.
Note: cook it without fat.

Low-sugar breakfast cookie★★/*Biscuit pour petit-déjeuner allégé en sucre*: cookie adapted to breakfast, rich in cereals and low in sugar. Carbohydrate.

Low-sugar food★★/*Allégé en sucre*: a food containing a lower quantity of sugar than the original food.

Low-sugar jam/*Confiture allégée en sucre*: jam which sugar quantity is reduced compared to original jam.

Lucerne seed★★★/*Graine de luzerne*: alfalfa seed eaten crushed or germinated.

Lumpfish roe★★★/*Œuf de lumps*: red or black fish eggs.

Lupin flour★★★/*Farine de lupin*: powder made of lupin seeds milling. Gluten-free.

Lupin milk★★★/*Lait de lupin*: plant milk from lupin seeds. Lactose-free.
Note: do not consume if it's sweetened.

Lupin milk cream dessert/*Crème dessert au lait de lupin*: vegetable dessert made of lupin milk, sugar and eggs. Dairy product.

Lychee in light syrup/*Litchi au sirop léger*: poached lychee preserved in more or less sugary water. Exotic fruit.

Lychee in syrup/*Litchi au sirop*: poached lychee preserved in very sugary water. Exotic fruit.

Lychee juice★/*Jus de litchi*: juice made of the pressing of lychees. Exotic fruit.

M

Maasdam cheese★/*Maasdam*: hard cow's milk cheese.
Note: do not consume more than approximately ½ oz of cheese three times per week... and never at dinner.

Macadamia nut/*Noix de macadamia*: cf. "Nut".

Macadamia nut spread/*Pâte à tartiner de noix de macadamia*: very sugary and fat mix of crushed macadamia nuts.

Macaroni★★★/*Macaroni*: hard wheat semolina pasta in the shape of a tube. Carbohydrate.

Macaroon/*Macaron*: small soft round cake made of almonds, white eggs and sugar.

Macchiato★★★/*Café noisette*: coffee with a drop of milk.
Note: do not consume if it's sweetened.

Mace★★★/*Macis*: capsule and peel of the nutmeg used as a condiment.

Macédoine★★★/*Macédoine*: mix of green vegetables or fruits cut in pieces.

Mackerel in muscadet wine★★★/*Maquereau au muscadet*: preserved mackerel fillets marinated in muscadet wine.

Mackerel in white wine★★★/*Maquereau au vin blanc*: preserved mackerel fillets marinated in dry white wine.

Mackerel rillettes★★/*Rillettes de maquereau*: cooked meat made of mackerel cooked in vegetable oil.

Mackerel with escabeche sauce★★★/*Maquereau à la sauce escabèche*: mackerel fillets preserved in escabeche sauce.

Mackerel with lemon★★★/*Maquereau au citron*: mackerel fillets preserved in lemon.

Mackerel with mustard sauce★★★/*Maquereau à la moutarde*: mackerel fillets preserved in mustard sauce.

Mackerel with tomato sauce★★★/*Maquereau à la sauce tomate*: mackerel fillets preserved in tomato sauce.

Madeira wine★/*Madère*: fortified wine.
Note: do not drink alcoholic beverage, however no problem if it's cooked.

Madeira wine sauce★★/*Sauce madère*: sauce made of flour, butter, lardons, stock and Madeira wine.

Madeleine/*Madeleine*: small cake in the shape of a bulging shell.

Malted yeast★★★/Levure maltée: yeast made of barley malt.

Mandarin in light syrup/*Mandarine au sirop léger*: poached mandarin preserved in more or less sugary water.

Mandarin in syrup/*Mandarine au sirop*: poached mandarin preserved in very sugary water.

Mandarin juice★/*Jus de mandarine*: juice made of the pressing of mandarins.

Mango in light syrup/*Mangue au sirop léger*: poached mango preserved in more or less sugary water. Exotic fruit.

Mango in syrup/*Mangue au sirop*: poached mango preserved in very sugary water. Exotic fruit.

Mango juice★/*Jus de mangue*: juice made of the pressing of mangoes. Exotic fruit.

Maple syrup/*Sirop d'érable*: sweetened solution made from the evaporation of the sugar maple sap.

Maranta arundinacea★★★/*Arrow-root*: starch of Maranta root. Gluten-free.

Mare's milk/*Lait de jument*: whole milk produced by mares.

Margarine★★/*Margarine*: plant-based dietary fats.
Note: consume it in moderation. Do not cook with it.

Marinade★★★/*Marinade*: liquid aromatic mix made of vinegar, salt, spices, etc. in which meat or fish macerates.

Mariniere (mussels)★★★/*Marinière (moules à la)*: mussels cooked in dry white wine with onions and herbs.

Marinière sauce★★★/*Sauce marinière*: white sauce made of fish stock and white wine.

Marmalade/*Marmelade*: mashed fruits previously cut in pieces and cooked with sugar until they become a purée.

Maroilles cheese★/*Maroilles*: soft raw cow's milk cheese with washed rind. Dairy product.
Note: do not consume more than approximately ½ oz of cheese three times per week... and never at dinner.

Marshmallow(1)/*Guimauve*: candy with a squishy consistency made of mallow root.

Marshmallow(2)/*Marshmallow*: soft marshmallow coated with powdered sugar and starch.

Mascarpone/*Mascarpone*: very creamy and fresh Italian cheese made of cow's milk. Dairy product.

Maté★★★/*Maté*: herbal tea made of roasted American holly leaves.
Note: do not consume if it's sweetened.

Mayonnaise/*Mayonnaise*: cold sauce made of an emulsion of egg yolks, mustard and oil.

Mead/*Hydromel*: alcoholic beverage made of honey fermented in water.

Meagre★★★/*Maigre*: saltwater fish with white flesh.
Note: cook it without fat: en papillote, in water, grill, roast...

Meat extracts★★★/*Extraits de viande*: beef or poultry meat concentrate in small packet or in cube (like KUB OR).

Meat jelly★/*Gelée de viande*: cleared and hardened meat juice.

Meat juice★/*Jus de viande*: juice made thanks to the cooking of a meat or of a poultry.

Meatloaf★/*Pain de viande*: dish made of potatoes, meat, butter and eggs served cold with a mayonnaise.

Meatloaf pâté en croûte★★/*Pâté de viande en croûte*: dish made of ground meat wrapped in puff pastry. Cooked meat.

Medlar in light syrup/*Nèfle au sirop léger*: poached medlar preserved in more or less sugary water.

Medlar in syrup/*Nèfle au sirop*: poached medlar preserved in very sugary water.

Melon in light syrup/*Melon au sirop léger*: poached melon preserved in more or less sugary water.

Melon in syrup/*Melon au sirop*: poached melon preserved in very sugary water.

Melted cheese★/*Fromage fondu*: cheese made of one or two cheese which have been melted. Dairy product. American cheese, cup cheese, Philadelphia
Note: do not consume more than approximately ½ oz of cheese three times per week... and never at dinner.

**Merguez★/*Merguez*: fresh spicy sausage made of beef or beef and mutton. Cooked meat.
Note: cook it without fat: to grill, to roast, etc.

**Meringue/*Meringue*: light pastry made of whipped egg whites and sugar baked in the oven.

**Mesclun★★★/*Mesclun*: mix of various young salads and aromatic plants. Green vegetable.

**Mesembryanthemum crystallinum★★★/*Ficoïde glaciale*: vegetable plant from which we eat the leaves. Green vegetable.

**Mexican sauce★★★/*Sauce mexicaine*: sauce made of tomatoes, bell peppers, onions and spices.

**Milanese (fish)/*Milanaise (poisson à la)*: fish which has been breaded with an egg before being fried.

**Milanese (meat)/*Milanaise (viande à la)*: meat which has been breaded with an egg before being fried.

**Milk chocolate/*Chocolat au lait*: cocoa powder mixed with sugar and butter or other things (or not)...

**Milk in tube/*Lait en tube*: cf. "Sweetened concentrated milk".

**Milk roll/*Pain au lait*: viennoiserie.

**Mille-feuille/*Mille-feuille*: puff pastry cake stuffed with pastry cream.

**Millet flake★★★/*Flocon de millet*: small portion of dehydrated millet. Carbohydrate. Gluten-free.

**Millet milk★★★/*Lait de millet*: plant milk from millets. Lactose-free.
Note: do not consume if it's sweetened.

Millet milk cream dessert/*Crème dessert au lait de millet*: vegetable dessert made of millet milk, sugar and eggs. Dairy product.

Millet pasta★★★/*Pâte alimentaire de millet*: mix to be cooked made of refined millet flour. Carbohydrate. Gluten-free.

Milliasse★★★/*Milliasse*: mash made of sieved corn flour before being cooled and grilled. Carbohydrate. Gluten-free.

Mimolette cheese★/*Mimolette*: hard cow's milk cheese. Dairy product.
Note: do not consume more than approximately ½ oz of cheese three times per week... and never at dinner.

Miner's lettuce: cf. "Claytonia perfoliata".

Minestrone★★/*Minestrone*: soup made of vegetables and lard with pasta or rice.

Mint★★★/*Menthe*: aromatic plant used as a condiment.

Mirabelle plum in light syrup/*Mirabelle au sirop léger*: poached mirabelle plum preserved in more or less sugary water.

Mirabelle plum in syrup/*Mirabelle au sirop*: poached mirabelle plum preserved in very sugary water.

Miso★★★/*Miso*: traditional Japanese dish made of fermented soybean paste.

Mixed vegetables★★★/*Jardinière de légumes*: mix of various green vegetables and carbohydrates cut in small pieces.

Mocha cake/*Moka*: cake made of a genoise stuffed with a butter cream flavored with coffee.

Mombins in light syrup/*Mombin au sirop léger*: poached mombins preserved in more or less sugary water. Exotic fruit.

Mombins in syrup/*Mombin au sirop*: poached mombins preserved in very sugary water. Exotic fruit.

Monkey bread★★/*Pain de singe*: fruit from the baobab tree. Exotic fruit.

Monosodium glutamate★★★/*Glutamate monosodique*: glutamate sodium used as a flavor enhancer.

Monterey Jack cheese★: pasteurised cow's milk cheese. Dairy product.
Note: do not consume more than approximately ½ oz of cheese three times per week... and never at dinner.

Morbier cheese★/*Morbier*: pressed raw cow's milk cheese. Dairy product.
Note: do not consume more than approximately ½ oz of cheese three times per week... and never at dinner.

Mornay sauce★★/*Sauce Mornay*: white sauce to which grated gruyère is added.

Morsel★★/*Bouchée*: puff pastry stuffed with various food compositions, example: bouchée à la reine.
Note: do not consume if it's sweetened.

Moussaka★★★/*Moussaka*: dish made of alternating layers of eggplant, ground mutton and thick béchamel baked in the oven.
Note: to cook béchamel only with olive oil, no with butter.

Mousseline/*Mousseline*: very light mashed potatoes. Carbohydrate.

Mozzarella★★/*Mozzarella*: soft cow's milk cheese, sometimes made with buffalo's milk. Dairy product.

Muenster cheese★: pasteurised cow's milk cheese. Dairy product.
Note: do not consume more than approximately ½ oz of cheese three times per week... and never at dinner.

Muesli with dark chocolate/*Muesli au chocolat noir*: mix of cereal flakes and dark chocolate curls. Carbohydrate.

Muesli with dried fruits/*Muesli aux fruits secs*: mix of cereal flakes and dried fruits. Carbohydrate.

Muesli with milk chocolate/*Muesli au chocolat au lait*: mix of cereal flakes and milk chocolate curls. Carbohydrate.

Muesli with nuts/*Muesli aux noix*: mix of cereal flakes and various nuts. Carbohydrate.

Muffin(1)★★/*Muffin(1)*: small plain white bread with leaven. Carbohydrate.

Muffin(2) /*Muffin(2)*: small round cake often containing fruits, sometimes with chocolate.

Mulberries in light syrup/*Mulberries au sirop léger*: poached mulberries preserved in more or less sugary water.

Mulberries in syrup/*Mulberries au sirop*: poached mulberries preserved in very sugary water.

Mullet★★★/*Mulet*: saltwater and freshwater fish with white flesh.
Note: cook it without fat: en papillote, in water, grill, roast...

Multi-grain bread/*Pain multicéréale*: cf. "Wholewheat bread". Carbohydrate.

Multivitamin juice - Myrciaria in syrup

Multivitamin juice★/*Jus multivitaminé*: mix of fruit juices, mainly apple and orange juices.

Mung bean/*Haricot mungo*: cf. "Soy bean".

Mung bean sprout★★★/*Pousse de haricot mungo*: young mung bean sprouts. Green vegetable.

Munster cheese★/*Munster*: soft cow's milk cheese with washed rind. Dairy product.
Note: do not consume more than approximately ½ oz of cheese three times per week... and never at dinner.

Mushroom in brine★★★/*Champignon en saumure*: sterilized mushroom in its salty cooking water. Green vegetable.

Mushroom sauce★★★/*Sauce champignon*: sauce made of tomatoes, onions, mushrooms and herbs.

Mushroom stock★★★/*Fumet de champignon*: very reduced stock made of mushrooms.

Mussel★★★/*Moule*: edible mollusk.

Mustard★★★/*Moutarde*: condiment made of mustard seeds and vinegar.

Mustard seed★★★/*Graine de moutarde*: mustard seed eaten crushed or germinated.

Myrciaria in light syrup/*Camu-camu au sirop léger*: poached myrciaria preserved in more or less sugary water. Exotic fruit.

Myrciaria in syrup/*Camu-camu au sirop*: poached myrciaria preserved in very sugary water. Exotic fruit.

N

Nattō★★★/*Nattō*: fermented soy bean sprouts.

Natural apple/*Pomme au naturel*: cf. "Fresh apple".

Natural apricot/*Abricot au naturel*: cf. "Fresh apricot".

Natural aronia/*Aronia au naturel* : cf. "Fresh aronia".

Natural azerole/*Azerole au naturel*: cf. "Fresh azerole".

Natural blackberry/*Mûre au naturel*: cf. "Fresh blackberry".

Natural blackcurrant/*Cassis au naturel*: cf. "Fresh blackcurrant".

Natural button mangosteen/*Mangoustan au naturel*: cf. "Fresh button mangosteen".

Natural carambola/*Carambole au naturel*: cf. "Fresh carambola".

Natural cherimoya/*Anone au naturel*: cf. "Fresh cherimoya".

Natural cherry/*Cerise au naturel*: cf. "Fresh cherry".

Natural clementine/*Clémentine au naturel*: cf. "Fresh clementine".

Natural cranberry/*Canneberge au naturel*: cf. "Fresh cranberry".

Natural fruit cocktail - Natural mombins

Natural fruit cocktail★★★**/***Cocktail de fruit au naturel*: mix of various fruits cut in dices and preserved in their juice without anything else added.

Natural grapefruit/*Pamplemousse au naturel*: cf. "Fresh grapefruit".

Natural guava/*Goyave au naturel*: cf. "Fresh guava".

Natural jujube/*Jujube au naturel*: cf. "Fresh jujube". Exotic fruit.

Natural kaki/*Kaki au naturel*: cf. "Fresh kaki".

Natural kiwi/*Kiwi au naturel*: cf. "Fresh kiwi".

Natural kumquat/*Kumquat au naturel*: cf. "Fresh kumquat".

Natural lemon/*Citron au naturel*: cf. "Fresh lemon".

Natural longan/*Longane au naturel*: cf. "Fresh longan".

Natural lychee/*Litchi au naturel*: cf. "Fresh lychee".

Natural mandarin/*Mandarine au naturel*: cf. "Fresh mandarin".

Natural mango/*Mangue au naturel*: cf. "Fresh mango".

Natural medlar/*Nèfle au naturel*: cf. "Fresh medlar".

Natural melon/*Melon au naturel*: cf. "Fresh melon".

Natural mirabelle plum/*Mirabelle au naturel*: cf. "Fresh mirabelle plum".

Natural mombins/*Mombin au naturel*: cf. "Fresh mombins".

**Natural mulberries/*Mulberries au naturel*: cf. "Fresh mulberries".

**Natural mushroom★★★/*Champignon au naturel*: sterilized mushroom in its unsalted cooking water. Green vegetable.

**Natural myrciaria dubia/*Camu-camu au naturel*: cf. "Fresh myrciaria dubia".

**Natural nectarine/*Brugnon au naturel*: cf. "Fresh nectarine".

**Natural olive★★/*Olive au naturel*: fresh olive sterilized in unsalted water.

**Natural orange/*Orange au naturel*: cf. "Fresh orange".

**Natural papaya/*Papaye au naturel*: cf. "Fresh papaya".

**Natural passion fruit/*Grenadille au naturel*: cf. "Fresh passion fruit".

**Natural peach/*Pêche au naturel*: cf. "Fresh peach".

**Natural pear/*Poire au naturel*: cf. "Fresh pear".

**Natural pineapple/*Ananas au naturel*: cf. "Fresh pineapple".

**Natural plum/*Prune au naturel*: cf. "Fresh plum".

**Natural quince/*Coing au naturel*: cf. "Fresh quince".

**Natural rambutan/*Ramboutan au naturel*: cf. "Fresh rambutan".

**Natural redcurrant/*Groseille au naturel*: cf. "Fresh redcurrant".

Natural salak - Navy beans with tomato sauce

Natural salak/*Salacca au naturel*: cf. "Fresh salak".

Natural salmon★★★/*Saumon au naturel*: salmon in a can without anything else except for salt.

Natural sapodilla fruit/*Sapotille au naturel*: cf. "Fresh sapodilla fruit".

Natural sardine★★★/*Sardine au naturel*: sardine preserved without adding anything nor transforming it, expect for sterilization.

Natural sloe/*Prunelle au naturel*: cf. "Fresh sloe".

Natural sorb/*Sorbe au naturel*: cf. "Fresh sorb".

Natural sweet wine/*Vin doux naturel*: wine fortified thanks to the adding of alcohol during its alcoholic fermentation.

Natural tamarind fruit/*Tamarin au naturel*: cf. "Fresh tamarind".

Natural tuna★★★/*Thon au naturel*: tuna in a can without anything else except for salt.

Natural watermelon/*Pastèque au naturel*: cf. "Fresh watermelon".

Nature knuckle of ham★★★/*Jambonneau nature*: part of the leg above the knee.

Nature shoyu★★★/*Shoyu nature*: fermented soy bean sauce.

Navy bean★★★/*Haricot blanc*: white or white and black bean seed eaten fully ripe. Carbohydrate.

Navy beans with tomato sauce★★★/*Haricots blancs sauce tomate*: navy beans cooked in tomato sauce.

Neapolitan sauce★★★/*Sauce napolitaine*: sauce made of tomatoes, olives and various aromatic herbs.

Nectarine/*Nectarine*: cf. "Peach".

Nectarine in light syrup/*Brugnon au sirop léger*: poached nectarine preserved in more or less sugary water.

Nectarine in syrup/*Brugnon au sirop*: poached nectarine preserved in very sugary water.

Nettle★★★/*Ortie*: herbaceous plant from which we eat the leaves. Green vegetable.

Neufchâtel cheese★/*Neufchâtel*: soft cow's milk cheese with bloomy rind. Dairy product.
Note: do not consume more than approximately ½ oz of cheese three times per week... and never at dinner.

New Zealand spinach★★★/*Tétragone*: vegetable plant from which we eat the leaves. Green vegetable.

Ninespine stickleback★★★/*Epinochette*: small freshwater fish with white flesh.
Note: cook it without fat: en papillote, grill. Do not fry.

Niolo★/*Niolo*: goat or sheep milk cheese. Dairy product.
Note: do not consume more than approximately ½ oz of cheese three times per week... and never at dinner.

Noisette potato★★★/*Pomme noisette*: dish in the shape of a small ball made of mashed potatoes and flour before being fried and baked in the oven. Carbohydrate.

Nori★★★/*Nori*: edible seaweed.

Nougat/*Nougat*: confection made of a mix of sugar, honey, egg whites, almonds, hazelnuts and pistachios.

Nuoc-mâm sauce★★★/*Sauce nuoc-mâm*: putrefied anchovy extract.

Nutmeg★★★/*Noix de muscade*: fruit from the myristica fragrans which grated seed is used as a condiment.

Nutsedge flake★★★/*Flocon de souchet*: small portion of dehydrated nutsedge. Carbohydrate.

Nutsedge flour★★★/*Farine de souchet*: powder made of nutsedge milling. Gluten-free.

O

Oat bran★★★/*Son d'avoine*: residue of oat milling.

Oat cream★★★/*Crème d'avoine*: more or less liquid cream made of oat milk, substitute to crème fraîche.

Oat flake★★★/*Flocon d'avoine*: small portion of dehydrated oats. Carbohydrate.

Oatmeal★★★/*Porridge*: oats mush. Carbohydrate.
Note: do not consume if it's sweetened.

Oat milk★★★/*Lait d'avoine*: plant milk from oats. Lactose-free.
Note: do not consume if it's sweetened.

Oat milk cream dessert/*Crème dessert au lait d'avoine*: vegetable dessert made of oat milk, sugar and eggs. Dairy product.

Oat pasta★★★/*Pâte alimentaire à base d'avoine*: mix to be cooked made of refined oat flour. Carbohydrate.

Oats★★★/*Avoine*: cereal which seeds are edible. Carbohydrate.

Octopus★★★/*Poulpe*: octopus from which we eat the tentacles.
Note: cook it without fat: en papillote, in water, grill, roast...

Œuf au lait/*Œuf au lait*: dessert made of eggs, milk and sugar.

Offals/*Abats*: edible part of meat animals that is not flesh nor muscles: kidney, liver, tongue, trotter, lungs, blood and black sausage... (See each offal separately in this book).

Okra★★★/*Gombo*: tropical green vegetable.

Oleaginous fruit/*Fruit oléagineux*: fruit rich in fats, most of the time, it consists in seeds: almonds, nuts, avocados, etc. See each of them depending on their own name.

Olive à la grecque★★/*Olive à la grecque*: olive preserved in a mixture rich in salt and in various spices.

Olive in brine★★/*Olive en saumure*: fresh olive sterilized in salted water.

Olivet cheese★/*Olivet*: soft cow's milk cheese with washed rind. Dairy product.
Note: do not consume more than approximately ½ oz of cheese three times per week... and never at dinner.

100% pure juice freshly pressed fruit juice (any fruit)★/*Jus de fruit 100% pur jus fraîchement pressé (tous fruits confondus)*: juice made of the pressing of fruits, without adding any sugar or additive (colorant, flavor, preserver...) and drunk immediately.

100% pure juice freshly pressed vegetable juice (any green vegetable)★★★/*Jus de légume 100% pur jus fraîchement pressé (tous légumes verts confondus)*: juice of green vegetables made of the

**100% pure juice industrial fruit juice
- 100% whole-grain einkorn wheat pasta**

pressing of vegetables, without adding anything and drunk immediately.

100% pure juice industrial fruit juice (any fruit)★/*Jus de fruit 100% pur jus industriel (tous fruits confondus)*: fruit juice industrially made of the pressing of fruits, without adding any sugar or additive (colorant, flavor, preserver...).

100% pure juice industrial vegetable juice (any green vegetable)★★★/*Jus de légume 100% pur jus industriel (tous légumes verts confondus)*: juice of green vegetables industrially made of the pressing of vegetables without adding anything.

100% whole-grain almond pasta★★★/*Pâte alimentaire à base d'amande complet*: mix to be cooked made of whole-grain almond flour. Gluten-free.

100% whole-grain amaranth pasta★★★/*Pâte alimentaire à base d'amarante complet*: mix to be cooked made of whole-grain amaranth flour. Gluten-free.

100% whole-grain barley pasta★★★/*Pâte alimentaire d'orge complet*: mix to be cooked made of whole-grain barley flour. Carbohydrate.

100% whole-grain buckwheat pasta★★★/*Pâte alimentaire de sarrasin complet*: mix to be cooked made of whole-grain buckwheat flour. Carbohydrate.

100% whole-grain corn pasta★★★/*Pâte alimentaire de maïs complet*: mix to be cooked made of whole-grain corn flour. Carbohydrate. Gluten-free.

100% whole-grain einkorn wheat pasta★★★/*Pâte alimentaire de petit épeautre complet*: mix to be cooked made of whole-grain einkorn wheat flour. Carbohydrate.

100% whole-grain findi pasta★★★/*Pâte alimentaire de fonio complet* : mix to be cooked made of whole-grain findi flour. Carbohydrate. Gluten-free.

100% whole-grain khorasan wheat pasta★★★/*Pâte alimentaire de kamut complet*: mix to be cooked made of whole-grain khorasan wheat. Carbohydrate.

100% whole-grain millet pasta★★★/*Pâte alimentaire de millet compet*: mix to be cooked made of whole-grain millet flour. Carbohydrate. Gluten-free.

100% whole-grain oat pasta★★★/*Pâte alimentaire à base d'avoine compet*: mix to be cooked made of whole-grain oat flour. Carbohydrate.

100% whole-grain quinoa pasta★★★/*Pâte alimentaire de quinoa complet*: mix to be cooked made of whole-grain quinoa flour. Carbohydrate. Gluten-free.

100% whole-grain rice pasta★★★/*Pâte alimentaire de riz complet*: mix to be cooked made of whole-grain rice flour. Carbohydrate. Gluten-free.

100% whole-grain rye pasta★★★/*Pâte alimentaire de seigle complet*: mix to be cooked made of whole-grain rye flour. Carbohydrate.

100% whole-grain soybean pasta★★★/*Pâte alimentaire de soja complet*: mix to be cooked made of whole-grain soybean flour. Carbohydrate. Gluten-free.

100% whole-grain spelt pasta★★★/*Pâte alimentaire d'épeautre complet*: mix to be cooked made of whole-grain spelt flour. Carbohydrate.

100% wholewheat pasta★★★/*Pâte alimentaire de blé complet*: mix to be cooked made of wholewheat semolina. Carbohydrate.

Omelet★★★/*Omelette*: dish made of beaten eggs cooked in a frying pan.

Onion★★★/*Oignon*: vegetable plant from which we eat the bulb. Green vegetable.

Onion salt★★★/*Sel d'oignon*: mix of table salt and dehydrated onion in powder.

Onion sausage★/*Saucisse à l'oignon*: ground pork flesh seasoned with onions, etc. before being put in a casing made of intestines. Cooked meat.
Note: cook it without fat: to grill, to roast, etc.

Onion seed★★★/*Graine d'oignon*: onion seed eaten crushed or germinated.

Oolong tea★★★/*Thé oolong*: tea between green tea and black tea.
Note: do not consume if it's sweetened.

Orangeade/Orangeade: beverage made of orange juice, sugar and water.

Orange in light syrup/*Orange au sirop léger*: poached orange preserved in more or less sugary water.

Orange in syrup/*Orange au sirop*: poached orange preserved in very sugary water.

Orange juice★/*Jus d'orange*: juice made of the pressing of oranges.

Orange roughy★★★/*Empereur*: saltwater fish with white flesh.
Note: cook it without fat: en papillote, in water, grill, roast...

Oregano★★★/*Origan*: aromatic plant used as a condiment.

Oriental borage★★★/*Bourrache orientale*: plant used as a condiment and from which we eat the young leaves.

Orzo★★★/*Café d'orge*: drink made of roasted barley malt.
Note: do not consume if it's sweetened.

Ossau-Iraty★/*Ossau-Iraty*: pressed sheep milk cheese.
Note: do not consume more than approximately ½ oz of cheese three times per week... and never at dinner.

Osso buco★★★/*Osso-buco*: knuckle of veal cut in slices, stir-fried and cooked in a mixture made of dry white wine, onions and tomatoes.

Ostrich★★★/*Autruche*: big bird living in Africa and in the Middle-East.
Note: cook it without fat: en papillote, in water, grill, roast...

Outside flat cut★★/*Gîte à la noix*: posterior part of the leg of beef. Red meat.
Note: do not consume more than approximately 4 oz of red meat twice per week. Cook it without fat: en papillote, in water, grill, roast...

Oven fries★★★/*Frites au four*: pre-cooked potatoes baked in the oven. Carbohydrate. Gluten-free.

Oxalis tuberosa★★★/*Oca du Pérou*: vegetable plant from which we eat the tubers. Green vegetable.

Ox tripe★★★/*Gras-double*: tripe shop product made of beef rumen. Offal.

Oyster★★★/*Huître*: edible mollusk.

Oyster sauce★★★/*Sauce d'huître*: sauce made of oyster stock reduction with corn starch.

$\mathcal{P}$

Paddy rice/*Riz paddy*: cf. "Whole-grain rice".

Paella★★★/*Paella*: Spanish dish made of rice flavored with saffron, browned in oil and cooked in stock, with meat, fish, crustacea, etc.

Pain au chocolat/*Pain au chocolat*: pastry stuffed with a chocolate bar.

Pain aux raisins/*Pain aux raisins*: viennoiserie made of raisins and custard.

Pain de Gênes/*Pain de Gênes*: viennoiserie made of cookie dough in which crushed almonds are put.

Paleleaved: cf. "Helianthus strumosus".

Palm heart★★★/*Cœur de palmier*: edible heart of palm in light brine.

Palm oil★★/*Huile de palme*: fatty substance made of palm kernel.

Palm oil-free margarine★★★/*Margarine sans huile de palme*: palm oil-free plant-based dietary fats.
Note: consume it in moderation. Do not cook with it.

Pancakes★★★/*Pancakes*: small thick crepes made of sieved flour. Carbohydrate.
Note: do not consume if it's sweetened.

Pancetta/*Pancetta*: Italian cooked meat made of salted pork breast which has been rolled and dried.

Panettone/*Panettone*: brioche stuffed with dried and candied fruits. Carbohydrate.

Panna cotta/*Panna cotta*: dessert made of milk, sugar, crème fraîche and gelatin.

Papaya in light syrup/*Papaye au sirop léger*: poached papaya preserved in more or less sugary water. Exotic fruit.

Papaya in syrup/*Papaye au sirop*: poached papaya preserved in very sugary water. Exotic fruit.

Papaya juice★/*Jus de papaye*: juice made of the pressing of papayas. Exotic fruit.

Paprika★★★/*Paprika*: sweet chili pepper in powder.

Paraffin oil★★★/*Huile de paraffine*: vegetable oil that is not assimilated by your metabolism.

Parmesan cheese★/*Parmesan*: hard Italian cheese made of cow's milk. Dairy product.
Note: do not consume more than approximately ½ oz of cheese three times per week... and never at dinner.

Parsley★★★/Persil: vegetable plant used as a condiment. Green vegetable.

Parsley juice★★★/*Jus de persil*: juice made of the pressing of parsley.

Parsley seed★★★/*Graine de persil*: parsley seed eaten crushed or germinated.

Parsnip★★★/*Panais*: vegetable plant grown for its edible root. Green vegetable.

Parsnip chips/*Chips de panais*: very thinly cut parsnip, fried and salted.

Partridge★★★/*Perdrix*: edible and very appreciated bird. Game.
Note: cook it without fat: en papillote, in water, grill, roast...

Passion fruit in light syrup/*Grenadille au sirop léger*: poached passion fruit preserved in more or less sugary water. Exotic fruit.

Passion fruit in syrup/*Grenadille au sirop*: poached passion fruit preserved in very sugary water. Exotic fruit.

Passion fruit juice★/Jus de fruit de la passion: juice made of the pressing of passion fruits. Exotic fruit.

Pasteurized milk★★★/*Lait pasteurisé*: milk which has been thermally treated between 160°F and 185°F during 15 seconds before being rapidly cooled.
Note: do not drink whole milk.

Paupiette★★★/*Paupiette*: slice of meat stuffed with stuffing wrapped around itself. Made of pork, turkey or veal.

Pea milk★★★/*Lait de pois*: plant milk from peas. Lactose-free.
Note: do not consume if it's sweetened.

Pea milk cream dessert/*Crème dessert au lait de pois*: vegetable dessert made of pea milk, sugar and eggs. Dairy product.

Peach in light syrup/*Pêche au sirop léger*: poached peach preserved in more or less sugary water.

Peach in syrup/Pêche au sirop: poached peach preserved in very sugary water.

Peach juice★/*Jus de pêche*: juice made of the pressing of peaches.

Peanut★/*Cacahuète*: roasted seed of the peanut plant.

Peanut butter/*Beurre de cacahuète*: peanut mixed with sugar.

Peanut flour★★/*Farine d'arachide*: powder made of not wholewheat peanut milling. Gluten-free.

Peanut milk★★/*Lait d'arachide*: plant milk from peanuts. Lactose-free.
Note: do not consume if it's sweetened.

Peanut oil★★/Huile d'arachide: fatty substance made of peanut.

Peanut purée★/Purée d'arachide: mashed peanut seeds to spread.

Pear in light syrup/*Poire au sirop léger*: poached pear preserved in more or less sugary water.

Pear in syrup/*Poire au sirop*: poached pear preserved in very sugary water.

Pear juice★/*Jus de poire*: juice made of the pressing of pears.

Pecan nut/*Noix de pécan*: cf. "Nut".

Peking duck★★/*Laqué (canard)*: duck which has been coated with sweet and sour sauce between two cookings.

Pecking pork★★/*Laqué (porc)*: pork which has been coated with sweet and sour sauce between two cookings.

Pepino dulce★★★/*Poire-melon*: annual vegetable plant producing this fruit.

Pepper★★★/*Poivre*: greatly savory and spicy spice.

Pepper sauce - Physalis peruviana

Pepper sauce/*Sauce au poivre*: sauce made with flour and butter with milled pepper.

Perch★★★/*Perche*: freshwater fish with white flesh.
Note: cook it without fat: en papillote, in water, grill, roast...

Pesto★★/*Pesto*: mix of ground basil, garlic, grated parmesan cheese and olive oil.
Note: do not consume more than approximately ½ oz of cheese three times per week... and never at dinner.

Pesto sauce★★/*Sauce pesto*: sauce made of tomatoes, basils and parmesan cheese.
Note: do not consume more than approximately ½ oz of cheese three times per week... and never at dinner.

Petit four/*Petit-four*: small pastry the size of a morsel, made of a dry pastry or stuffed with cream.

Petit suisse★★★/*Petit-suisse*: fromage frais in cylindrical shape. Dairy product.
Note: the less fat, the better!

Petit suisse flavored with fruits★/*Petit-suisse aromatisé aux fruits*: sweetened fromage frais in cylindrical shape with fruits. Dairy product.
Note: the less fat, the better!

Pheasant★★★/*Faisan*: gallinaceous bird valued for its flesh. Game.
Note: cook it without fat: en papillote, in water, grill, roast...

Philadelphia cheese★: pasteurised cow's milk cheese. Dairy product.
Note: do not consume more than approximately ½ oz of cheese three times per week... and never at dinner.

Physalis peruviana★★★/*Coqueret du Pérou*: vegetable plant from which we eat the berries.

Pickle★★★/*Cornichon*: kind of cucumber harvested young or very young and preserved in vinegar or brine. Green vegetable.

Pickles★★★/*Pickles*: small vegetables or fruits preserved in vinegar.

Pickleweed★★★/*Salicorne*: plant found on sea shores and from which we eat the stems as a condiment. Green vegetable.

Picodon★/*Picodon*: soft raw goat milk cheese.
Note: do not consume more than approximately ½ oz of cheese three times per week... and never at dinner.

Pie★★/*Tarte*: dish made of a thick pie garnished with cream, fish, meat, etc. before being baked in the oven.
Note: the less fat, the better!

Pie crust★★★/*Pâte brisée*: crust made of flour, butter and eggs. Carbohydrate.

Pig's ear★★/*Oreille de cochon*: pork's ear. Offal.

Pigeon★★★/*Pigeon*: small edible bird. Game.
Note: cook it without fat: en papillote, in water, grill, roast...

Pike★★★/*Brochet*: freshwater fish with white flesh.
Note: cook it without fat: en papillote, in water, grill, roast...

Pineapple in light syrup/*Ananas au sirop léger*: poached pineapple preserved in more or less sugary water. Exotic fruit.

Pineapple in syrup/*Ananas au sirop*: poached pineapple preserved in very sugary water. Exotic fruit.

Pineapple juice★/*Jus d'ananas*: juice made of the pressing of pineapples. Exotic fruit.

Pine kernel - Plaice

Pine kernel★★★/*Pignon de pin*: crushed pine kernel.

Pink grapefruit juice★/*Jus de pamplemousse rose*: juice made of the pressing of pink grapefruits.

Pinto bean★★★/*Haricot rosé*: cooked pinky seed eaten fully ripe. Carbohydrate.

Piperade★★★/*Piperade*: dish made of bell pepper, tomatoes and eggs.

Pistachio★/*Pistache*: seed from the pistachio tree.

Pistachio cream★★/*Crème de pistache*: pistachio spread.

Pistachio milk★★★/*Lait de pistache*: plant milk from pistachios. Lactose-free.
Note: do not consume if it's sweetened.

Pistachio milk cream dessert/*Crème dessert au lait de pistache*: vegetable dessert made of pistachio milk, sugar and eggs. Dairy product.

Pistachio purée★/*Purée de pistache*: mashed pistachios to spread.

Pitta★★/*Pita*: small unleavened white bread. Carbohydrate.

Pizza★/*Pizza*: bread dough galette covered with tomato sauce and various garnishes before being baked in the pizza oven. Carbohydrate.
Note: the less fat, the better!

Pizza base★★★/*Pâte à pizza*: base made of flour, water and yeast.

Plaice★★★/*Carrelet*: flat saltwater fish with white flesh.
Note: cook it without fat: en papillote, in water, grill, roast...

Plain breast bacon★/*Lard de poitrine nature*: plain piece of pork breast.

Plain cookie/*Biscuit sec*: cookie made of flour, sugar, eggs and fats.

Plain lardon★/*Lardon nature*: small piece of plain bacon used to prepare a dish.

Plain skimmed cow's milk yogurt★★★/*Yaourt au lait de vache maigre nature*: cow's milk which has been partially or completely skimmed before being fermented thanks to lactic acid bacteria, unsweetened. Dairy product.

Plain skimmed goat milk yogurt★★★/*Yaourt au lait de chèvre maigre nature*: goat milk which has been partially or completely skimmed before being fermented thanks to lactic acid bacteria, unsweetened. Dairy product.

Plain skimmed sheep milk yogurt★★★/*Yaourt au lait de brebis maigre nature*: sheep milk which has been partially or completely skimmed before being fermented thanks to lactic acid bacteria, unsweetened. Dairy product.

Plain sweetened whole cow's milk yogurt/*Yaourt au lait de vache entier nature sucré*: whole cow's milk fermented thanks to lactic acid bacteria before being sweetened. Dairy product.

Plain whole cow's milk yogurt★/*Yaourt au lait de vache entier nature*: whole cow's milk fermented thanks to lactic acid bacteria, unsweetened. Dairy product.

Plain whole goat milk yogurt★/*Yaourt au lait de chèvre entier nature*: whole goat milk fermented thanks to lactic acid bacteria, unsweetened. Dairy product.

Plain whole sheep milk yogurt - Porgy

Plain whole sheep milk yogurt★/*Yaourt au lait de brebis entier nature*: whole sheep milk fermented thanks to lactic acid bacteria, unsweetened. Dairy product.

Plantain★★★/*Banane plantain*: tropical fruit of the banana tree, rich in starch and eaten cooked. Exotic fruit.

Planter's punch/Planteur: punch made of rum, cane sugar and fruit juice.

Plant milk/*Lait végétal*: milk from various vegetables. All are lactose-free. See each plant milk separately.

Plum in light syrup/*Prune au sirop léger*: poached plum preserved in more or less sugary water.

Plum in syrup/*Prune au sirop*: poached plum preserved in very sugary water.

Polenta(1)★★★/*Polenta(1)*: chestnut mush. Gluten-free.

Polenta(2)★ ★★/*Polenta(2)*: corn mush. Gluten-free.

Pont-L'évêque cheese★/*Pont-L'évêque*: soft cow's milk with washed rind. Dairy product.
Note: do not consume more than approximately ½ oz of cheese three times per week… and never at dinner.

Popcorn/*Maïs pop corn*: puffed up corn kernel more or less sweetened. Gluten-free.

Poppy seed★★★/*Graine de pavot*: poppy seed eaten crushed.

Poppyseed oil★★/*Huile d'œillette*: fatty substance made of poppy seeds.

Porgy★★★/*Sar*: saltwater fish with white flesh.
Note: cook it without fat: en papillote, in water, grill, roast…

Pork (meat...)/*Porc (viande de...)*: all unprepared nor transformed meats, plain, ready to be cooked and cut from pork. See each piece separately.

Pork breast★/*Poitrine de porc*: inferior part of the pork's rib cage to boil.
Note: cook it without fat: grill, roast...

Pork chop★★★/*Côte de porc*: anterior part of the pork.
Note: cook it without fat: grill, roast...

Pork confit/*Confit de porc*: pork cooked and preserved in its cooking fat.

Pork hotpot★★/*Potée*: dish made of pork meat and boiled cabbage.

Pork kidney★★★/*Rognon de porc*: kidney of the pork. Offal.
Note: cook it without fat: grill, roast...

Pork liver★★★/*Foie de porc*: offal.
Note: cook it without fat: grill, roast...

Pork liver pâté/*Pâté de foie de porc*: minced pork liver cooked before being put in a baking pan. Cooked meat.

Pork loin(1)★ ★★/*Echine de porc*: anterior part of the pork.
Note: cook it without fat: grill, roast...

Pork loin(2)★★★/*Longe de porc*: pork meat corresponding to the upper part of the cervical and lumbar areas.
Note: cook it without fat: en papillote, in water, grill, roast...

Pork loin(3)★★★/*Rouelle de porc*: thick slice of pork leg.
Note: cook it without fat: en papillote, in water, grill, roast...

Pork rillettes - Potato flakes purée

Pork rillettes/*Rillettes de porc*: cooked meat made of pork meat cooked in its fat.

Pork shoulder★★★/*Palette de porc*: pork shoulder blade and the flesh around it.
Note: cook it without fat: en papillote, in water, grill, roast...

Pork spare ribs★★★/*Carré de porc*: piece of pork meat to roast or to grill.
Note: cook it without fat: grill, roast...

Pork tongue★★★/*Langue de porc*: pork tongue eaten boiled. Offal.
Note: cook it without fat.

Porridge★★★/*Bouillie*: doughy dish made of boiled flour and milk, or water. Carbohydrate.

Port salut★/*Port-salut*: pressed cow's milk cheese with washed rind. Dairy product.
Note: do not consume more than approximately ½ oz of cheese three times per week... and never at dinner.

Port wine/*Porto*: liqueur wine.

Potato★★★/*Pomme de terre*: vegetable plant from which we eat the tubers. Carbohydrate. Gluten-free.

Potatoes chips/*Chips de pomme de terre*: very thinly cut potatoes, fried and salted.

Potato flake/*Flocon de pommes de terre*: small portion of dehydrated potato, to make purée. Carbohydrate. Gluten-free.

Potato flakes purée/*Purée de pomme de terre en flocon*: dehydrated industrial mashed potatoes.

Potato starch★★★/*Fécule de pomme de terre*: starch from potatoes transformed into flour. Carbohydrate. Gluten-free.

Pot-au-feu★/*Pot-au-feu*: dish made of boiled beef meat, carrots, leeks, cabbage... Red meat.

Poulette sauce★★/*Sauce poulette*: white sauce with egg yolks and lemon juice.

Pouligny Saint-Pierre cheese★/*Pouligny Saint-Pierre*: raw goat milk cheese in the shape of a pyramid.
Note: do not consume more than approximately ½ oz of cheese three times per week... and never at dinner.

Poultry/*Volaille*: bird raised in barnyard such as hens, chickens, ducks, guinea fowls, gooses etc. See each poultry separately.

Poultry liver★★★/*Foie de volaille*: chicken, hen, duck, goose, etc. offal.
Note: cook it without fat or with olive oil.

Poultry liver pâté/*Pâté de foie de volaille*: minced poultry liver cooked before being put in a baking pan. Cooked meat.

Poultry quenelle★★★/*Quenelle de volaille*: poultry stuffing thickened with eggs and bread crumb before being shaped in the form of a sausage.

Poultry sausage★★★/*Saucisse de volaille*: sausage made of poultry meat. Cooked meat.
Note: cook it without fat.

Poultry stock★★★/*Fond de volaille*: brown stock made of poultry stock.

Pout★★★/*Tacaud*: saltwater fish with white flesh.
Note: cook it without fat: en papillote, in water, grill, roast...

Powder of dehydrated broth/*Bouillon déshydraté en poudre*: cf. "Cube of... broth".

Powder of myrciaria★★★/*Camu-camu en poudre*: extracts of myrciaria sold in capsules or in powder. Exotic fruit.

Powdered sugar/*Sucre glace*: white sugar in extremely thin powder. Fast-acting sugar.

Praline(1)/*Pralin*: mix of roasted and crushed hazelnuts and almonds with sugar.

Praline(2)/*Praliné*: mix of chocolate and crushed sugared almonds.

Preserve★★★/*Conserve*: sterilized food preserved in an airtight can.

Preserved plain grilled mackerel★★★/*Maquereau grillé nature en conserve*: preserved plain grilled mackerel fillets.

Pressed cooked cheese★/*Fromage à pâte pressée cuite*: beaufort cheese, comté cheese, emmental cheese, gruyère, parmesan cheese, capricious, Colby, Swiss cheese, Dry Jack... Dairy product.
Note: do not consume more than approximately ½ oz of cheese three times per week... and never at dinner.

Pressed uncooked cheese★/*Fromage à pâte pressée non cuite*: appenzeller cheese, cantal cheese, cheddar, édam cheese, Humboldt fog...
Note: do not consume more than approximately ½ oz of cheese three times per week... and never at dinner.

Pretzel/*Bretzel*: cookie into an 8-shape, sprinkled with salt and cumin.

Prickly pear★★/*Figue de Barbarie*: plump fruit from the opuntia (cactus).

Prickly pear juice★/*Jus de figue de Barbarie*: juice made of the pressing of prickly pears.

Prime rib of beef★★/*Côte de bœuf*: piece of beef meat to grill.
Note: do not consume more than approximately 4 oz of red meat twice per week.

Provel cheese★: pasteurised cow's milk cheese. Dairy product.
Note: do not consume more than approximately ½ oz of cheese three times per week... and never at dinner.

Provençale sauce★★★/*Sauce provençale*: sauce made of tomatoes, onions, bell peppers, olives, olive oil and thyme.

Provolone★/*Provolone*: cow's milk cheese which has been salted, dried and smoked. Dairy product.
Note: do not consume more than approximately ½ oz of cheese three times per week... and never at dinner.

Prune★/*Pruneau*: plum which has been dried in the oven or to the sun.

Prune juice★/*Jus de pruneau*: juice made of the pressing of prunes.

Pudding/*Pudding*: sugary dessert made of bread crumb, semolina or rice, plain cookie, eggs, crème fraîche and dried fruits.

Puffed barley pancake★★/*Galette d'orge soufflée*: extruded barley pancake. Carbohydrate. Gluten-free.
Note: do not consume if it's sweetened.

Puffed buckwheat pancake★★/*Galette de sarrasin soufflé*: extruded buckwheat pancake. Carbohydrate.
Note: do not consume if it's sweetened.

Puffed chocolate rice pancake
- Puffed rice pancake

Puffed chocolate rice pancake/*Galette de riz soufflé au chocolat*: extruded white rice pancake coated with chocolate. Gluten-free.

Puffed corn pancake★★/*Galette de maïs soufflé*: extruded corn pancake. Carbohydrate. Gluten-free.
Note: do not consume if it's sweetened.

Puffed einkorn wheat pancake★★/*Galette de petit épeautre soufflé*: extruded einkorn wheat pancake. Carbohydrate.
Note: do not consume if it's sweetened.

Puffed einkorn whole-grain pancake★★/*Galette de petit épeautre complet soufflé*: extruded whole-grain einkorn wheat pancake. Carbohydrate.
Note: do not consume if it's sweetened.

Puffed khorasan wheat pancake★★/*Galette de kamut soufflé*: extruded khorasan wheat pancake. Carbohydrate. Gluten-free.
Note: do not consume if it's sweetened.

Puffed millet pancake★★/*Galette de millet soufflé*: extruded millet pancake. Carbohydrate. Gluten-free.
Note: do not consume if it's sweetened.

Puffed oats pancake★★/*Galette d'avoine soufflée*: extruded oats pancake. Carbohydrate. Gluten-free.
Note: do not consume if it's sweetened.

Puffed quinoa pancake★★/*Galette de quinoa soufflé*: extruded quinoa pancake. Carbohydrate.
Note: do not consume if it's sweetened.

Puffed rice pancake★★/*Galette de riz soufflé*: extruded rice pancake. Carbohydrate. Gluten-free.
Note: do not consume if it's sweetened.

Puffed rye pancake★★/*Galette de seigle soufflé*:
extruded rye pancake. Carbohydrate. Gluten-free.
Note: do not consume if it's sweetened.

Puffed soybean pancake★★/*Galette de soja soufflé*:
extruded soybean pancake. Carbohydrate. Gluten-free.
Note: do not consume if it's sweetened.

**Puffed spelt pancake★★/*Galette d'épeautre
soufflé***: extruded spelt pancake. Carbohydrate.
Note: do not consume if it's sweetened.

**Puffed whole-grain barley pancake★★/*Galette
d'orge complète soufflée***: extruded whole-grain barley
pancake. Carbohydrate. Gluten-free.
Note: do not consume if it's sweetened.

**Puffed whole-grain buckwheat pancake
★★/*Galette de sarrasin complet soufflé***: extruded
whole-grain buckwheat pancake. Carbohydrate.
Note: do not consume if it's sweetened.

**Puffed whole-grain corn pancake★★/*Galette de
maïs complet soufflé***: extruded whole-grain corn
pancake. Carbohydrate. Gluten-free.
Note: do not consume if it's sweetened.

**Puffed whole-grain khorasan wheat
pancake★★/*Galette de kamut complet soufflé***:
extruded whole-grain khorasan wheat pancake.
Carbohydrate. Gluten-free.
Note: do not consume if it's sweetened.

**Puffed whole-grain millet pancake★★/*Galette de
millet complet soufflé***: extruded whole-grain millet
pancake. Carbohydrate. Gluten-free.
Note: do not consume if it's sweetened.

**Puffed whole-grain oats pancake
- Pumpkin seed flour**

Puffed whole-grain oats pancake★★/*Galette d'avoine complète soufflée*: extruded whole-grain oat pancake. Carbohydrate. Gluten-free.
Note: do not consume if it's sweetened.

Puffed whole-grain rice pancake★★/*Galette de riz complet soufflé*: extruded whole-grain rice pancake. Carbohydrate. Gluten-free.
Note: do not consume if it's sweetened.

Puffed whole-grain rye pancake★★/*Galette de seigle complet soufflé*: extruded whole-grain rye pancake. Carbohydrate. Gluten-free.
Note: do not consume if it's sweetened.

Puffed whole-grain soybean pancake★★/*Galette de soja complet soufflé*: extruded whole-grain soybean pancake. Carbohydrate. Gluten-free.
Note: do not consume if it's sweetened.

Puffed whole-grain spelt pancake★★/*Galette d'épeautre complet soufflé*: extruded whole-grain spelt pancake. Carbohydrate.
Note: do not consume if it's sweetened.

Puff pastry★★/*Pâte feuilletée*: pastry made of flour, butter and eggs. Carbohydrate.

Pulp-free fruit juice★/*Jus de fruit sans pulpe*: 100% pure juice fruit juice without the pulp.

Pumpkin(1)★★★/*Citrouille*: kind of squash, very big autumn fruit. Green vegetable.

Pumpkin(2)★★★/*Potiron*: vegetable plant from which we eat the fruit. Green vegetable.

Pumpkin seed flour★★★/*Farine de pépin de courge*: powder from pumpkin seed milling. Gluten-free.

Punch/*Punch*: alcoholic beverage made of rum and fruit juice.

Purée★★/*Purée*: dish made of mashed green vegetables or some mashed carbohydrates.

Purslane★★★/*Pourpier*: plant from which we eat the leaves in salad. Green vegetable.

Purslane seed★★★/*Graine de pourpier*: purslane seed eaten crushed or germinated.

Q

Quail★★★/*Caille*: small migratory bird close to the partridge. Game.
Note: cook it without fat: en papillote, in water, grill, roast...

Queen coris pâté/*Pâte de tamarin*: pressed and concentrated queen coris.

Quiche★★/*Quiche*: salted pie made of pie crust and garnished with lardons covered with flan mixture: eggs and crème fraîche.
Note: the less fat, the better!

Quince in light syrup/*Coing au sirop léger*: poached quince preserved in more or less sugary water.

Quince in syrup/*Coing au sirop*: poached quince preserved in very sugary water.

Quince jelly/*Pâte de coing*: confection made of quinces cooked in sugar.

Quinoa★★★/*Quinoa*: plant from which we eat the seeds. Carbohydrate. Gluten-free.

Quinoa cornflakes★★/*Corn flakes de quinoa*: grilled flakes made of quinoa flour. Carbohydrate. Gluten-free.
Note: do not consume if it's sweetened.

Quinoa cream★★★/*Crème de quinoa*: more or less liquid cream made of quinoa milk, substitute to crème fraîche.

Quinoa flake★★★/*Flocon de quinoa*: small portion of dehydrated quinoa. Carbohydrate. Gluten-free.

Quinoa flour★★★/*Farine de quinoa*: powder made of not whole-grain quinoa seed milling. Carbohydrate. Gluten-free.

Quinoa milk★★★/*Lait de quinoa*: plant milk from quinoa. Lactose-free.
Note: do not consume if it's sweetened.

Quinoa milk cream dessert/*Crème dessert au lait de quinoa*: vegetable dessert made of quinoa milk, sugar and eggs. Dairy product.

Quinoa pasta★★★/*Pâte alimentaire de quinoa*: mix to be cooked made of refined quinoa flour. Carbohydrate. Gluten-free.

Quinoa seed★★★/*Graine de quinoa*: quinoa seed eaten crushed or germinated.

Quinoa tabbouleh★★★/*Taboulé de quinoa*: mix of quinoa, tomatoes, onions, bell peppers, raisins and mint leaves with olive oil. Carbohydrate. Gluten-free.

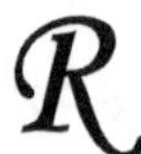

Rabbit terrine/Pâté de lapin: minced rabbit meat cooked before being put in a baking pan. Cooked meat.

Rabbit★★★/*Lapin*: herbivore mammal.
Note: cook it without fat: en papillote, in water, grill, roast...

Raclette(1)★/*Raclette(1)*: cow's milk cheese eaten melted. Dairy product.
Note: do not consume more than approximately ½ oz of cheese three times per week... and never at dinner.

Raclette(2) /*Raclette(2)*: dish made of raclette cheese, potatoes and various cooked meats.

Radish★★★/*Radis*: vegetable plant from which we eat the plump root. Green vegetable.

Raisin/*Raisin sec*: fruit from the vine which has been greatly dried.

Ramaria aurea★★★/*Clavaire doré*: mushroom you can find in the woods. Green vegetable.

Rambutan in light syrup/*Ramboutan au sirop léger*: poached rambutan preserved in more or less sugary water. Exotic fruit.

Rambutan in syrup/*Ramboutan au sirop*: poached rambutan preserved in very sugary water. Exotic fruit.

Rampion bellflower★★★/*Raiponce cultivée*: vegetable plant grown for its leaves and its roots eaten in salad. Green vegetable.

Rare (cooking)★★/*Saignante (cuisson)*: to not completely cook beef, duck or lamb. Red meat.
Note: do not consume more than approximately 4 oz of red meat twice per week. Cook it without fat: en papillote, in water, grill, roast...

Raspberry juice★/*Jus de framboise*: juice made of the pressing of raspberries.

**Ratatouille -
Ready-to-use flour for wholewheat bread**

Ratatouille★★★/**_Ratatouille_**: dish made of eggplants, bell peppers, tomatoes and zucchinis.

Raviole★★/**_Raviole_**: small square of pasta stuffed with cheese. Carbohydrate.
Note: do not consume more than approximately ½ oz of cheese three times per week... and never at dinner.

Raw (raw milk, raw meat, raw fish...)★★/**_Cru (lait cru, viande crue, poisson cru...)_**: food eaten without being previously cooked.

Raw milk★★★/**_Lait cru_**: milk from animals not thermally treated nor filtered.
Note: do not drink whole milk.

Raw milk cheese★/**_Fromage au lait cru_**: cheese made of milk that did not go under any heat treatment. Dairy product.
Note: do not consume more than approximately ½ oz of cheese three times per week... and never at dinner.

Razor clam★★★/**_Couteau_**: sea mollusk with a long shell.
Note: cook it without fat or with olive oil.

Ready-cooked dishes from the caterer★★/**_Plat cuisiné du traiteur_** : various dishes sold vacuum packed, frozen or fresh, made by an artisan from catering profession and ready to be eaten.

Ready-to-use flour for cereal bread★★★/**_Farine pour pain aux céréales prête à l'emploi_**: whole-grain cereal flour with seeds and salt.

Ready-to-use flour for white bread★★/**_Farine pour pain blanc prête à l'emploi_**: salted sieved cereal flour.

Ready-to-use flour for wholewheat bread★★★/**_Farine pour pain complet prête à l'emploi_**: salted whole-grain cereal flour.

Reblochon★/*Reblochon*: pressed raw cow's milk cheese with a washed rind. Dairy product.
Note: do not consume more than approximately ½ oz of cheese three times per week... and never at dinner.

Red ascophyllum★★★/*Goémon rouge*: edible seaweed.

Red berries fruit★/*Jus de fruits rouges*: juice made of the pressing of red berries.

Redcurrant in light syrup/*Groseille au sirop léger*: poached redcurrant preserved in more or less sugary water.

Redcurrant in syrup/*Groseille au sirop*: poached redcurrant preserved in very sugary water.

Red hawk cheese★: pasteurised cow's milk cheese. Dairy product.
Note: do not consume more than approximately ½ oz of cheese three times per week... and never at dinner.

Red kuri squash★★★/*Potimarron*: squash which taste is similar to that of the chestnut. Green vegetable.

Red Leicester cheese★: raw or pasteurised cow's milk cheese. Dairy product.

Red meat★★/*Viande rouge*: beef, lamb and horse meat.
Note: do not consume more than approximately 4 oz of red meat twice per week. Cook it without fat: en papillote, in water, grill, roast...

Red mullet★★★/*Rouget*: saltwater fish with white flesh.
Note: cook it without fat: en papillote, in water, grill, roast...

Red rice★★★/*Riz rouge*: rare red whole-grain rice.

Red sea bream★★★/*Rousseau*: saltwater fish with white flesh.
Note: cook it without fat: en papillote, in water, grill, roast...

Red wine★/*Vin rouge*: wine made thanks to the alcoholic fermentation of black grapes under the action of yeasts.
Note: do not drink alcoholic beverage, however no problem if it's cooked.

Red windsor★:   pasteurised cow's milk cheese. Dairy product.
Note: do not consume more than approximately ½ oz of cheese three times per week... and never at dinner.

Red yeast rice★★★/*Levure de riz rouge*: microscopic mushrooms grown on rice.

Reindeer milk/*Lait de renne*: whole milk produced by reindeers.

Remoulade sauce★★/*Sauce rémoulade*: sauce made of vegetable oil, mustard and shallots.

Rhubarb★★★/*Rhubarbe*: vegetable plant from which we eat the chards after cooking. Green vegetable.

Rib steak★★/*Entrecôte*: slice of beef cut between the ribs. Red meat.
Note: do not consume more than approximately 4 oz of red meat twice per week. Cook it without fat: en papillote, in water, grill, roast...

Rice bran★★★/*Son de riz*: residue of rice milling.

Rice bran oil★★/*Huile de riz*: fatty substance made of rice.

Rice bulgur★★★/*Boulgour de riz*: crushed white rice steamed or cooked in water. Carbohydrate. Gluten-free.

Rice cornflakes★★/*Corn flakes de riz*: grilled flakes made of white rice flakes. Carbohydrate. Gluten-free.
Note: do not consume if it's sweetened.

Rice cream★★★/*Crème de riz*: more or less liquid cream made of rice milk, substitute to crème fraîche.

Rice flake★★★/*Flocon de riz*: small portion of dehydrated rice. Carbohydrate. Gluten-free.

Rice flour★★★/*Farine de riz*: powder made of white rice milling. Carbohydrate. Gluten-free.

Rice milk★★★/*Lait de riz*: plant milk from rice. Lactose-free.
Note: do not consume if it's sweetened.

Rice milk cream dessert/*Crème dessert au lait de riz*: vegetable dessert made of rice milk, sugar and eggs. Dairy product.

Rice milk yogurt★★★/*Yaourt au lait de riz*: rice milk fermented thanks to lactic acid bacteria, sweetened or not. Dairy product. Lactose-free.
Note: do not consume if it's sweetened.

Rice pasta★★★/*Pâte alimentaire de riz*: mix to be cooked made of refined rice flour. Carbohydrate. Gluten-free.

Rice syrup/*Sirop de riz*: sweetener made from the fermentation of grain of rice and barley.

Ricotta★★/*Ricotta*: Italian cheese made of other cheese serum. Dairy product.

Rigotte★/*Rigotte*: raw goat milk cheese and raw cow's milk cheese. Dairy product.
Note: do not consume more than approximately ½ oz of cheese three times per week... and never at dinner.

Rind/*Couenne*: pork skin.

Rind (cheese)★/*Croûte (du fromage)*: external part of the cheese.

Risotto★★/*Risotto*: rice cooked in broth with onions and various other foods.

Roach★★★/*Gardon*: freshwater fish with white flesh.
Note: cook it without fat: to grill, to roast, etc.

Roast★★★/*Rôti*: piece of meat or of poultry baked in the oven.
Note: cook it without fat.

Roast beef★★/*Rosbif*: piece of roasted beef. Red meat.
Note: do not consume more than approximately 4 oz of red meat twice per week. Cook it without fat.

Roasted spelt★★★/*Epeautre torréfié*: roasted beverage similar to coffee.
Note: do not consume if it's sweetened.

Rocamadour cheese★/*Rocamadour*: round and flat cheese made of raw goat milk. Dairy product.
Note: do not consume more than approximately ½ oz of cheese three times per week... and never at dinner.

Rockfish★★★/*Sébaste*: saltwater fish with white flesh.
Note: cook it without fat: en papillote, in water, grill, roast...

Rognonnade★★★/*Rognonnade*: veal loin rolled and garnished with kidneys. Offal.

Rollmops★★★/*Rollmops*: raw herring rolled around a pickle marinated in vinegar and spices.

Rollot★★/*Rollot*: soft cow's milk cheese in the shape of a heart. Dairy product.
Note: do not consume more than approximately ½ oz of cheese three times per week... and never at dinner.

Romanesco broccoli★★★/*Chou romanesco*: cabbage from which we eat the central inflorescence.

Rond de tranche★/*Rond de tranche*: fat and very tender piece of beef corresponding to quadriceps. Red meat.
Note: do not consume more than approximately 4 oz of red meat twice per week. Cook it without fat: en papillote, in water, grill, roast...

Rooster/*Coq*: cf. "Hen". Poultry.

Roquefort★/*Roquefort*: raw sheep milk cheese with parsley in it. Dairy product.
Note: do not consume more than approximately ½ oz of cheese three times per week... and never at dinner.

Rose hip★★★/*Cynorhodon*: berry from the dog rose eaten as jam.

Rosemary★★★/*Romarin*: aromatic plant.

Rosé wine/*Vin rosé*: pink wine.

Roux★★/*Roux*: mix of flour and fat used to thicken sauces.
Note: to made without butter but with olive oil.

Royal jelly★★★/*Gelée royale*: liquid secreted by nurse bees.

Ruffe★★★/*Grémille*: small freshwater with white flesh.
Note: cook it without fat: grill...

Rum★/*Rhum*: eau de vie made from sugar cane juice distillation.
Note: do not drink alcoholic beverage, however no problem if it's cooked.

Rum baba/*Baba*: yeast cake with raisins and soaked with rum or Kirsch after cooking.

Rump steak★★/*Rumsteck*: tender piece of beef to grill or to roast. Red meat.
Note: do not consume more than approximately 4 oz of red meat twice per week. Cook it without fat: en papillote, in water, grill, roast...

Rutabaga★★★/*Rutabaga*: vegetable plant from which we eat the swollen root. Green vegetable.

Rye★★★/*Seigle*: cereal source of gluten from which flour is extracted. Carbohydrate.

Rye bread★★★/*Pain de seigle*: bread made of rye flour. Carbohydrate.

Rye flake★★★/*Flocon de seigle*: small portion of dehydrated rye. Carbohydrate.

Rye milk★★★/*Lait de seigle*: plant milk from rye. Lactose-free.
Note: do not consume if it's sweetened.

Rye milk cream dessert/*Crème dessert au lait de seigle*: vegetable dessert made of rye milk, sugar and eggs. Dairy product.

Rye pasta★★★/*Pâte alimentaire de seigle*: mix to be cooked made of refined rye flour. Carbohydrate.

S

Saccharine★★★/*Saccharine*: synthetic sweetener.

Saccharose/*Saccharose*: cf. "White sugar".

Safflower oil★★/*Huile de carthame*: fatty substance made of safflower.

Saffron★★★/*Safran*: spice.

Sage★★★/*Sauge*: plant used as a condiment.

Saint-André cheese★/*Saint-André*: soft cow's milk cheese with bloomy rind. Triple cream cheese. Dairy product.
Note: do not consume more than approximately ½ oz of cheese three times per week... and never at dinner.

Sainte-Maure★/*Sainte-Maure*: raw goat milk cheese in the shape of a long cylinder. Dairy product.
Note: do not consume more than approximately ½ oz of cheese three times per week... and never at dinner.

Saint-Félicien cheese/*Saint-Félicien*: cf. "Saint-Marcellin".

Saint-Florentin★/*Saint-Florentin*: soft raw or pasteurized cow's milk cheese with washed rind. Dairy product.
Note: do not consume more than approximately ½ oz of cheese three times per week... and never at dinner.

Saint Honoré cream/*Crème saint honoré*: cf. "Custard". Dairy product.

Saint-Marcellin★/*Saint-Marcellin*: soft cow's milk cheese with bloomy rind. Dairy product.
Note: do not consume more than approximately ½ oz of cheese three times per week... and never at dinner.

Saint-Nectaire★/*Saint-Nectaire*: pressed raw cow's milk cheese with bloomy rind. Dairy product.
Note: do not consume more than approximately ½ oz of cheese three times per week... and never at dinner.

Saint-Paulin cheese★/*Saint-Paulin*: pressed raw cow's milk cheese with washed rind. Dairy product.
Note: do not consume more than approximately ½ oz of cheese three times per week... and never at dinner.

Salad★★/*Salade*: leafy vegetable plant such as watercress, curly endive, lettuce, lamb's lettuce, etc. Green vegetable.

Salad burnet★★★/*Pimprenelle*: aromatic plant used as a condiment.

Salak in light syrup/*Salacca au sirop léger*: poached salak preserved in more or less sugary water. Exotic fruit.

Salak in syrup/*Salacca au sirop*: poached salak preserved in very sugary water. Exotic fruit.

Salami/*Salami*: Italian saucisson sec. Cooked meat.

Salers cheese★/*Salers*: pressed raw cow's milk cheese.
Note: do not consume more than approximately ½ oz of cheese three times per week... and never at dinner.

Salmis★★★/*Salmis*: stew made of game or poultry pieces cooked in a sauce made of red wine.

Salmon carpaccio★★★/*Carpaccio de saumon*: salmon flesh cut in very thin slices eaten raw, with a drop of olive oil and lemon juice.

Salmon quenelle★★★/*Quenelle de saumon*: salmon stuffing thickened with eggs and bread crumb before being shaped in the form of a sausage.

Salmon rillettes★★/*Rillettes de saumon*: cooked meat made of salmon cooked in vegetable oil.

Salsify★★★/*Salsifis*: vegetable plant from which we eat the root. Green vegetable.

Salt pork★/*Petit salé*: pork breast cooked in a flavored stock.
Note: cook it without fat: to grill, to roast, etc.

Salt pork with lentils★/*Petit salé aux lentilles*: dish cooked in sauce and made of pork breast and lentils.

Salt-free & gluten-free crispbread★★/*Biscotte sans sel & sans gluten*: slice of salt-free and gluten-free sandwich bread industrially toasted in the oven. Carbohydrate.

Salt-free cookie/*Biscuit sans sel*: cookie that does not contain salt. Carbohydrate.

Salt-free crispbread★★/*Biscotte sans sel*: slice of salt-free sandwich bread industrially toasted in the oven. Carbohydrate.

Salt-free grain bread★★★/*Pain aux céréales sans sel*: bread made of wholewheat flour with cereal grains with not salt in the batter during the kneading. Carbohydrate.

Salt-free margarine★★/*Margarine sans sel*: salt-free plant-based dietary fats.
Note: consume it in moderation. Do not cook with it.

Salt-free white bread★★/*Pain blanc sans sel*: bread made of sieved cereal flour with no salt in the batter during the kneading. Carbohydrate.

Salt-free wholewheat bread★★★/*Pain complet sans sel*: bread made of wholewheat flour with no salt in the batter during the kneading. Carbohydrate.

Salt substitute★★★/*Substitut de sel*: preparation without sodium chloride used as a substitute to salt.

Saltwater fish★★★/*Poisson marin*: every fatty and lean fish found in salted waters.
Note: cook it without fat: en papillote, in water, grill, roast...

Samosa★★/*Samoussa*: triangular fritter made of a thin flour dough wrapping a stuffing made of meat, fish, rice vermicelli, green vegetables, etc.

Sandwich★★/*Sandwich*: bread cut in slices between which you put a slice of meat, fish, cheese, etc.
Note: the less fat, the better!

Sandwich bread★/*Pain de mie*: white bread without crust. Carbohydrate.

Sapodilla fruit in light syrup/*Sapotille au sirop léger*: poached sapodilla fruit preserved in more or less sugary water. Exotic fruit.

Sapodilla fruit in syrup/*Sapotille au sirop*: poached sapodilla fruit preserved in very sugary water. Exotic fruit.

Sardine in chili pepper★★★/*Sardine au piment*: sardine preserved in oil and in chili pepper.

Sardine in herbes★★★/*Sardine aux herbes*: sardine preserved in oil and aromatic herbes.

Sardine in lemon★★★/*Sardine au citron*: sardine preserved in oil and lemon.

Sardine in oil★/*Sardine à l'huile*: sardine preserved in oil.

Sardine in tomato sauce★★★/*Sardine à la tomate*: sardine preserved in tomato sauce.

Sardinella★★★/*Sardinelle*: fatty saltwater fish.

Sardine rillettes★★/*Rillettes de sardine*: cooked meat made of sardine cooked in vegetable oil.

Sashimi★★★/*Sashimi*: dish made of raw fish and seafoods with soy sauce.

Sashimi sauce/*Sauce sashimi*: cf. "Sushi sauce".

Sauce gribiche★★/*Sauce gribiche*: sauce made of eggs, vegetable oil, pickles, vinegar and herbs.

Saucisson sec/*Saucisson sec*: big sausage eaten raw after desiccation. Cooked meat.

Sauerkraut(1)★★★/*Choucroute(1)*: fermented white cabbage.

Sauerkraut(2)★/*Choucroute(2)*: fermented white cabbage with cooked meats, pork meat and potatoes.

Sauté (cooking process)★★/*Sauté (cuisson en)*: to cook food in fat over an open fire.
Note: to cook only with olive oil.

Savory★★★/*Sarriette*: plant used as a condiment.

Savory cake/*Cake*: cake made of an egg batter with yeast, candied fruits and raisins soaked in rum.

Sbrinz★/*Sbrinz*: hard raw cow's milk which has been aged for a long time. Dairy product.
Note: do not consume more than approximately ½ oz of cheese three times per week... and never at dinner.

Scabbard fish★★★/*Sabre*: saltwater fish with white flesh.
Note: cook it without fat: en papillote, in water, grill, roast...

Scallion★★★/*Ciboule*: plant close to the garlic and from which we eat the bulging leaves.

Scallop★★★/*Coquille saint Jacques*: edible sea mollusk.
Note: cook it without fat except with olive oil.

Scolymus★★★/*Scolyme*: vegetable plant from which we eat the roots. Green vegetable.

Scorpion fish★★★/*Rascasse*: saltwater fish with white flesh.
Note: cook it without fat: en papillote, in water, grill, roast...

Scorzonera★★★/*Scorsonère*: vegetable plant from which we eat the long black roots. Green vegetable.

Scotch/*Scotch*: Scottish whiskey.

Scrambled egg★★★/*Œuf brouillé*: lightly cooked scrambled egg in an oiled frying pan.

Sculpin★★★/*Chabot*: freshwater fish with white flesh.
Note: cook it without fat: en papillote, in water, grill...

Sea bream★★★/*Daurade* : saltwater fish with white flesh.
Note: cook it without fat: en papillote, in water, grill, roast...

Seafood/*Fruit de mer*: edible crustacea and shellfish. See each of them depending on their own name.

Sea lettuce★★★/*Ulve*: edible seaweed. Green vegetable.

Sea trout★★★/*Truite de mer*: fatty saltwater fish.
Note: cook it without fat: en papillote, in water, grill, roast...

Sea urchin★★★/*Oursin*: very thorny saltwater animal.

Seaweed chips/*Chips d'algue*: cooked and compressed seaweeds very thinly cut before being fried and salted.

Seaweed mustard★★★/*Moutarde aux algues*: condiment made of mustard seeds, edible seaweeds and vinegar.

Seaweed tartare★★/*Tartare d'algue*: dish made of edible seaweeds, vegetable oil and various condiments.

Seeds★★★/*Graines*: mix of sunflower seeds, wheat seeds, barley seeds, sesame seeds, etc.

Seltz water★★★/*Eau de seltz*: water that is naturally or artificially fizzy.

Semi-skimmed cow's milk★★/*Lait de vache demi-écrémé*: milk produced by cows and which has been partially skimmed.

Semi-skimmed goat milk★★/*Lait de chèvre demi-écrémé*: goat milk which has been partially skimmed.

Semi-skimmed sheep milk★★/*Lait de brebis demi-écrémé*: sheep milk which has been partially skimmed.

Sepiola★★★/*Sépiole*: small edible cuttlefish.
Note: cook it without fat: en papillote, in water, grill, roast...

Serviceberry★★★/*Alise*: red fruit from the whitebeam.
Note: consume it immediately after the meal.

Sesame cream★★★/*Crème de sésame*: condiment made of crushed sesame seeds.

Sesame flour - Sheep milk cheese

Sesame flour★★★/***Farine de sésame***: powder made of sesame seeds milling. Gluten-free.

Sesame oil★★/***Huile de sésame***: fatty substance made of sesame seeds.

Sesame purée★★★/***Purée de sésame***: mashed sesame seeds to spread.

Sesame seed★★★/***Graine de sésame***: sesame seed eaten crushed.

Sesame seed milk★★★/***Lait de graines de sésame***: plant milk from sesame seeds. Lactose-free.
Note: do not consume if it's sweetened.

Sesame seeds milk cream dessert/*Crème dessert au lait de graines de sésame*: vegetable dessert made of sesame seed milk, sugar and eggs. Dairy product.

Shad★★★/***Alose***: fatty freshwater fish.
Note: cook it without fat: en papillote, in water, grill, roast...

Shallot★★★/***Echalote***: vegetable plant close to the onion and grown for its bulb. Green vegetable.

Shandy/*Panaché*: beverage made for half of beer and half of lemon soda.

Shashlik★★/***Chachlik***: goat meat skewered and marinated in spicy vinegar. Red meat.
Note: do not consume more than approximately 4 oz of red meat twice per week. Cook it without fat: en papillote, in water, grill, roast...

Sheep milk cheese★/***Fromage de brebis***: cheese made of sheep milk. Dairy product.
Note: do not consume more than approximately ½ oz of cheese three times per week... and never at dinner.

Sheep milk cottage cheese★★★/*Faisselle au lait de brebis*: fresh cheese made of sheep milk. Dairy product.
Note: the less fat, the better!

Sheep milk cream dessert/*Crème dessert au lait de brebis*: dairy specialty or dessert made of sheep milk, sugar and eggs. Dairy product.

Sheep milk fromage blanc★★★/*Fromage blanc de brebis*: fresh cheese made of sheep milk, a bit drained and not aged. Dairy product.
Note: the less fat, the better!

Shepherd's pie★★/*Hachis parmentier*: dish made of ground meat and mashed potatoes grilled into the oven.
Note: do not consume more than approximately 4 oz of red meat twice per week.

Sherry/*Xérès*: cf. "Vinegar".

Shiitake★★★/*Shiitake*: fresh or dried edible mushroom. Green vegetable.

Shin★★/*Gîte*: beef shank. Red meat.
Note: do not consume more than approximately 4 oz of red meat twice per week. Cook it without fat: en papillote, in water, grill, roast...

Shirred egg★★/*Œuf cocotte*: egg with crème fraîche baked in the oven in ramekins.

Shortbread biscuit/*Sablé*: small round biscuit made of sugar, egg yolks and butter.

Shoulder of beef★★/*Macreuse*: piece of beef made of the shoulder muscles to simmer or to boil. Red meat.
Note: do not consume more than approximately 4 oz of red meat twice per week. Cook it without fat.

Shoulder of lamb - Sium sisarum

Shoulder of lamb★★/*Epaule d'agneau*: tender and rather fat meat from the lamb. Red meat.
Note: do not consume more than approximately 4 oz of red meat twice per week. Cook it without fat: en papillote, in water, grill, roast...

Shoulder of veal★★★/*Epaule de veau*: tender meat to roast coming from the veal.
Note: cook it without fat: to grill, to roast, etc.

Shrimp★★★/*Crevette*: small sea crustacean.
Note: cook it without fat except with olive oil.

Shrimp chips/*Chips de crevette*: swelled chips made of tapioca and shrimp flours.

Shropshire cheese★: pasteurised cow's milk cheese. Dairy product.
Note: do not consume more than approximately ½ oz of cheese three times per week... and never at dinner.

Sichuan pepper★★★/*Poivre de Sichuan*: spice.

Silurid fish★★★/*Silure*: freshwater fish with white flesh.
Note: cook it without fat: en papillote, in water, grill, roast...

Sirloin★★/*Aloyau*: piece of beef meat consisting of the fillet, the sirloin and the rump steak. Red meat.
Note: do not consume more than approximately 4 oz of red meat twice per week. Cook it without fat: grill, roast...

Sirloin steak★★/*Faux-filet*: tasty but fat beef meat. Red meat.
Note: do not consume more than approximately 4 oz of red meat twice per week. Cook it without fat: grill, roast...

Sium sisarum★★★/*Chervis*: vegetable plant from which we eat the cooked roots. Green vegetable.

62% fat lightly salted butter★★/*Beurre demi-sel à 62% de matières grasses*: lightly salted butter which fat quantity has been reduced from one fourth compared to traditional butter.
Note: consume it in moderation. Do not cook with it.

62% fat lightly unsalted butter★★/*Beurre doux à 62% de matières grasses*: unsalted butter which fat quantity has been reduced from one fourth compared to traditional butter.
Note: consume it in moderation. Do not cook with it.

Skate (wing)★★★/*Raie (aile de)*: gristly saltwater fish. Fish with white flesh.
Note: cook it without fat: en papillote, in water, grill, roast...

Skimmed cow's milk★★★/*Lait de vache écrémé*: cow's milk which has been completely skimmed.

Skimmed goat milk★★★/*Lait de chèvre écrémé*: goat milk completely skimmed.

Skipjack tuna★★★/*Bonite*: fatty saltwater fish.
Note: cook it without fat: en papillote, in water, grill, roast...

Skirt steak★★/*Hampe de bœuf*: portion of the beef diaphragm. Red meat.
Note: do not consume more than approximately 4 oz of red meat twice per week. Cook it without fat: grill, roast...

Slice of fillet★★★/*Tranche de filet*: piece of pork meat to grill.
Note: cook it without fat: to grill, to roast, etc.

Slippery elm★★★/*Orme rouge*: powder made of slippery elm bark.

Sloe in light syrup/*Prunelle au sirop léger*: poached sloe preserved in more or less sugary water.

Sloe in syrup/*Prunelle au sirop*: poached sloe preserved in very sugary water.

Small pea★★★/*Petit pois*: round and green seed from the pea harvested fresh. Green vegetable.

Smelt★★★/*Eperlan* : saltwater fish with white flesh.
Note: cook it without fat: en papillote, in water, grill, roast...

Smoked breast bacon★/*Lard de poitrine fumé*: salted and smoked piece of pork breast.
Note: cook it without fat: to grill, to roast, etc.

Smoked fatty fish★★★/*Poisson gras fumé*: fatty fish which has been salted (more or less) and smoked.
Note: cook it without fat: en papillote, in water, grill, roast...

Smoked haddock★★★/*Haddock*: smoked haddock fish.
Note: cook it without fat: en papillote, grill, roast...

Smoked ham★★★/*Jambon fumé*: raw pork ham salted before being smoked. Cooked meat.
Note: cook it without fat: to grill, to roast, etc.

Smoked herring★★★/*Hareng fumé*: herring which went under a smoking process.
Note: cook it without fat: en papillote, grill, roast...

Smoked lardon★/*Lardon fumé*: small piece of salted and smoked bacon used to prepare a dish.

Smoked lean fish★★★/*Poisson maigre fumé*: lean fish which has been salted (more or less) and smoked.
Note: cook it without fat: to grill, to roast, etc.

Smoked meat★★★/*Viande fumée*: meat which has been salted before being smoked.
Note: cook it without fat: to grill, to roast, etc. Do not consume more than approximately 4 oz of red meat twice per week.

Smoked salmon★★★/*Saumon fumé*: salmon which has been salted before being smoked.

Smoked sausage★/*Saucisse fumée*: pork sausage which has been smoked. Cooked meat.
Note: cook it without fat: grill, roast...

Smoked trout★★★/*Truite fumée*: filet of salted and smoked trout.

Smoked vegetable ham★★★/*Jambon végétal fumé*: vegetarian product made of cereals and vegetable oil.

Snacking/*Grignotage*: to frequently eat small quantities of food.

Snails★★★/*Escargot*: small gastropod mollusk.
Note: to cook only with olive oil.

Snow pea★★★/*Pois mange-tout*: kind of peas from which we eat the clove and the seeds. Green vegetable.

Soda/*Soda*: fizzy beverage made of water, gas and sugar, or even fruit juice.

Soft-boiled egg★★★/*Œuf à la coque*: egg cooked in a lot of water without the egg yolk being completely cooked.
Note: do not consume more than 3 eggs per week.

Soft cheese with bloomy rind★/*Fromage à pâte molle et à croûte fleurie*: brie cheese, camembert, carré de l'Est, chaource cheese, coulommiers cheese, neufchâtel cheese, saint-marcellin, d'Isigny cheese... Dairy product.
Note: do not consume more than approximately ½ oz of cheese three times per week... and never at dinner.

**Soft cheese with washed rind
- Sorb preserved in light syrup**

Soft cheese with washed rind★/*Fromage à pâte molle et à croûte lavée*: époisses de Bourgogne, munster cheese, livarot cheese, maroilles cheese, olivet cendré, pont-l'évêque cheese, rollot cheese, saint-florentin cheese, soumaintrain cheese, vacherin cheese, Red hawk, Muenster, Teleme cheese, Brick cheese, lierderkrantz cheese... Dairy product.
Note: do not consume more than approximately ½ oz of cheese three times per week... and never at dinner.

Soft frik★★★/*Frik tendre*: crushed not fully grown hard wheat without its peel. Carbohydrate.

Soft pepper★★★/*Poivre doux*: not very savory and not very spicy spice.

Soft shell clam★★★/*Mye*: shellfish, edible saltwater mollusk.
Note: cook it without fat except with olive oil.

Sole★★★/*Sole*: flat saltwater fish with white flesh.
Note: cook it without fat: en papillote, in water, grill, roast...

Soluble coffee★★★/*Café soluble*: grains of dehydrated coffee.
Note: do not consume if it's sweetened.

Sorbet/*Sorbet*: frozen dessert made of sugar and fruit purée or fruit juice.

Sorbet-filled fruit/*Givré*: fruit which inside part is stuffed with sorbet.

Sorb in syrup/*Sorbe au sirop*: poached sorb preserved in very sugary water.

Sorb preserved in light syrup/*Sorbe au sirop léger*: poached sorb preserved in more or less sugary water.

Sorghum flake★★★/*Flocon de sorgho*: small portion of dehydrated sorghum. Carbohydrate.

Sorghum flour★★★/*Farine de sorgho*: powder made of sorghum milling. Carbohydrate. Gluten-free.

Sorghum pasta★★★/*Pâte alimentaire de sorgho*: mix to be cooked made of sorghum flour. Carbohydrate. Gluten-free.

Sorrel★★★/*Oseille*: vegetable plant with edible leaves. Green vegetable.

Soufflé★★★/*Soufflé*: dish made of whipped egg whites which, during the cooking process, increase the volume of the dish.

Soumaintrain★/*Soumaintrain*: soft cow's milk cheese with a washed rind. Dairy product.
Note: do not consume more than approximately ½ oz of cheese three times per week... and never at dinner.

Soursop★★/*Corossol*: fruit from the Annona muricata. Exotic fruit.

Soybean★★★/*Soja*: legume from which we eat the seeds.

Soy bean★★★/*Haricot de soja*: green soybean seed. Green vegetable.

Soybean flake★★★/*Flocon de soja*: small portion of dehydrated soybean. Carbohydrate.

Soybean flour★★★/*Farine de soja*: flour made of not whole-grain soybean milling. Gluten-free.

Soybean pasta★★★/*Pâte alimentaire de soja*: mix to be cooked made of refined soybean flour. Carbohydrate. Gluten-free.

Soy bean sprout★★★/*Germe de soja*: young sprout from the mung bean seed. Green vegetable.

Soybean vermicelli★★★/*Vermicelle chinois*: pasta made of soybean flour in the shape of long and thin filaments. Gluten-free.

Soy cream★★★/*Crème de soja*: more or less liquid cream made of soy milk, substitute to crème fraîche.

Soy milk★★★/*Lait de soja*: plant milk from soybean. Lactose-free.
Note: do not consume if it's sweetened.

Soy milk cream dessert/*Crème dessert au lait de soja*: vegetable dessert made of soy milk, sugar and eggs. Dairy product.

Soy milk fromage blanc★★★/*Fromage blanc de soja*: fresh cheese made of soy milk. Dairy product. Lactose-free.
Note: do not consume if it's sweetened.

Soy milk yogurt★★★/*Yaourt au lait de soja*: soy milk fermented thanks to lactic acid bacteria, sweetened or not. Dairy product. Lactose-free.
Note: do not consume if it's sweetened.

Soy oil★★/*Huile de soja*: fatty substance made of soybean.

Soy sauce★★★/*Sauce soja*: fermented vegetable proteins with meat flavors.

Spare rib★★/*Travers de porc*: extremity of pork ribs.
Note: cook it without fat: to grill, to roast, etc.

Sparkling wine/*Vin mousseux*: wine or cider containing carbon dioxide.

Speculaas/*Spéculoos*: very sugary plain cookie.

Spelt bulgur★★★/*Boulgour d'épeautre*: sieved and crushed spelt steamed or cooked in water. Carbohydrate.

Spelt coffee★★★/*Café d'épeautre*: spelt seeds drunk once roasted.
Note: do not consume if it's sweetened.

Spelt cornflakes★★/*Corn flakes d'épeautre*: grilled flakes made of sieved spelt flakes. Carbohydrate.
Note: do not consume if it's sweetened.

Spelt flake★★★/*Flocon d'épeautre*: small portion of dehydrated spelt. Carbohydrate.

Spelt milk★★★/*Lait d'épeautre*: plant milk from spelts. Lactose-free.
Note: do not consume if it's sweetened.

Spelt milk cream dessert/*Crème dessert au lait d'épeautre*: vegetable dessert made of spelt milk, sugar and eggs. Dairy product.

Spelt pasta★★★/*Pâte alimentaire d'épeautre*: mix to be cooked made of refined spelt flour. Carbohydrate.

Spices★★★/*Epices*: clove, chili pepper, turmeric, curry, etc.

Spider crab★★★/*Araignée*: sea crustacean looking like a crab.
Note: cook it without fat: en papillote, in wate ...

Spiky bitter melon★★★/*Margose à piquant*: vegetable plant from which we eat the green fruits. Green vegetable.

Spinach★★★/*Epinard*: vegetable plant from which we eat the long leaves. Green vegetable.

Spinach seed★★★/*Graine d'épinard*: spinach seed eaten crushed or germinated.

Spiny dogfish - Squash seed purée

Spiny dogfish★★★/*Aiguillat*: edible shark.
Note: cook it without fat: en papillote, in water, grill, roast...

Spirulina★★★/*Spiruline*: sea cyanobacteria used to make diet foods.

Spirulina pasta★★★/*Pâte alimentaire de spiruline*: mix to be cooked made of spirulina. Green vegetable.

Split pea★★★/*Pois cassé*: dried peas eaten in purée. Carbohydrate. Gluten-free.

Split pea flake★★★/*Flocon de pois cassés*: small portion of dehydrated split pea flakes. Carbohydrate. Gluten-free.

Split pea pasta★★★/*Pâte alimentaire de pois cassés*: mix to be cooked made of split pea flour. Carbohydrate. Gluten-free.

Spring roll★★/*Nem*: small rice flour crepe stuffed with meat, vegetables and rice vermicelli before being rolled and fried. Gluten-free.

Spring roll sauce/*Sauce pour nem*: cf. "Nuoc-mâm sauce".

Squash seed★★★/*Graine de courge*: grilled squash seed.

Squash seed oil★★/*Huile de pépin de courge*: fatty substance made of squash seeds.

Squash seed purée★★★/*Purée de graine de courge*: mashed squash seeds to spread.

Squid★★★**/*Calamar***: sea mollusk very appreciated for its flesh.
Note: cook it without fat: en papillote, in water, grill, roast...

Stachys affinis★★★**/*Crosne du Japon***: vegetable plant from which we eat the rhizomes. Green vegetable.

Standard olive oil★★**/*Huile d'olive standard***: fatty substance made of olive.

Star anise/*Anis étoilé*: cf. "Anise".

Steak tartare★★**/*Steak tartare***: ground beef steak eaten raw. Red meat.
Note: do not consume more than approximately 4 oz of red meat twice per week.

Steak/*Steak*: cf. "Beefsteak".

Steam★★★**/*Etouffée (à l')***: cooking method for meats and dried legumes with a very small quantity of liquid or even no liquid at all and a lid on.

Sterilized UHT heavy cream/*Crème entière stérilisée UHT*: fats from sterilized milk (30%) with which the butter is made. Made of sterilized UHT milk. Dairy product.

Stevia (extracts)★★★**/*Stévia (extraits de)***: very sugary extract of a plant called "Stevia", used as a sweetener instead of sugar, very low in calorie.

Stew(1)★★**/*Civet***: rabbit or other game stew marinated in red wine and cooked in a sauce thickened with blood. Game.
Note: cook it without fat except with olive oil.

Stew - Stock

Stew(2)★★/*Ragoût*: dish made of meat or fish cut in pieces and cooked in a sauce made of roux.
Note: to cook only with olive oil. Do not consume more than approximately 4 oz of red meat twice per week.

Stichelton cheese★: raw cow's milk cheese. Dairy product.
Note: do not consume more than approximately ½ oz of cheese three times per week... and never at dinner.

Stickleback★★★/*Epinoche*: small freshwater fish with white flesh.
Note: cook it without fat: en papillote, in water, to grill. Do not fry.

Still water★★★/*Eau plate*: natural water from the faucet or in bottle.

Stilton cheese★/*Stilton*: cow's milk cheese with pasteurized milk parsley in it. Dairy product.
Note: do not consume more than approximately ½ oz of cheese three times per week... and never at dinner.

Stinking bishop★: pasteurised cow's milk cheese. Dairy product.
Note: do not consume more than approximately ½ oz of cheese three times per week... and never at dinner.

Stir fry of cooked and frozen green vegetables★★/*Poêlée de légumes verts cuisinés surgelés*: green vegetables industrially cooked before being frozen and ready to be eaten.

Stir fry of uncooked frozen green vegetables★★★/*Poêlée de légumes verts non cuisinés surgelés*: plain green vegetables frozen, sold with their spices packet and ready to be eaten.

Stock★★★/*Court-bouillon*: flavored liquid in which you cook fish or meat.

Strawberry juice★/*Jus de fraise*: juice made of the pressing of strawberries.

Strudel/*Strudel*: pastry made of a rolled pastry stuffed with cinnamon apple and raisin.

Stuffed breakfast cookie/*Biscuit pour petit-déjeuner fourré*: stuffed cookie adapted to breakfast. Carbohydrate.

Stuffed olive★★/*Olive farcie*: olive stuffed with various condiments such as anchovies, bell peppers, etc.

Stuffing★★★/*Farce*: mix of mashed herbs, mashed vegetables, ground meat and crushed bread crumb put inside a poultry, a fish or a vegetable.

Sucralose★★★/*Sucralose*: sweetener used instead of sugar to get a sugary taste, very low in calorie.

Sugar cane/*Sucre de canne*: sugar only from cane sugar. Fast-acting sugar.

Sugared almond/*Dragée*: almond, chocolate or nut coated with sugar.

Sugar-free and salt-free cookie★★/*Gâteau sec sans sucre sans sel*: sugar-free but sweetened (in general with maltitol) cookie which contains a low quantity of salt or even no salt at all.

Sugar-free and semi-skimmed powder cow's milk★★/*Lait de vache demi-écrémé en poudre sans sucre*: dehydrated semi-skimmed cow's milk without added sugar.

Sugar-free and semi-skimmed powder goat milk★★/*Lait de chèvre demi-écrémé en poudre sans sucre*: dehydrated semi-skimmed goat milk without added sugar.

**Sugar-free and semi-skimmed powder sheep milk
- Sugar-free skimmed powder sheep milk**

Sugar-free and semi-skimmed powder sheep milk★★/*Lait de brebis demi-écrémé en poudre sans sucre*: dehydrated semi-skimmed sheep milk without added sugar.

Sugar-free cake★★/*Gâteau sans sucre*: pastry made of a sugar-free but sweetened batter, used alone or with a cream, fruits...

Sugar-free candy★★★/*Bonbon sans sucre*: candy only made of sweetener.

Sugar-free chewing gum★★★/*Chewing-gum sans sucre*: sweetened substance designed to be chewed.

Sugar-free chocolate spread★/*Pâte chocolatée à tartiner sans sucre*: sugar-free, but sweetened, and very fat mix of chocolate and crushed hazelnuts.

Sugar-free cookie★★/*Biscuit sans sucre*: sweetened cookie. Carbohydrate.

Sugar-free ketchup★★★/*Ketchup sans sucre*: thick spicy sauce made of tomatoes and sweetener.

Sugar-free plain muesli★★★/*Muesli nature sans sucre*: mix of cereal flakes without added sugar. Carbohydrate.

Sugar-free skimmed powder cow's milk★★★/*Lait de vache écrémé en poudre sans sucre*: dehydrated skimmed cow's milk without added sugar.

Sugar-free skimmed powder goat milk★★★/*Lait de chèvre écrémé en poudre sans sucre*: dehydrated skimmed goat milk without added sugar.

Sugar-free skimmed powder sheep milk★★★/*Lait de brebis écrémé en poudre sans sucre*: dehydrated skimmed sheep milk without added sugar.

**Sugar-free soda★★★/*Soda zéro*: fizzy beverage made of water, gas and one or several sweetener(s).

**Sugar-free whole cow's milk in powder/*Lait de vache entier en poudre sans sucre*: dehydrated whole cow's milk without added sugar.

**Sugar-free whole goat milk in powder/*Lait de chèvre entier en poudre sans sucre*: dehydrated whole goat milk without added sugar.

**Sugar-free whole sheep milk in powder/*Lait de brebis entier en poudre sans sucre*: dehydrated whole sheep milk without added sugar.

**Sumac★★★/*Sumac*: spice with a salty aftertaste.

**Sunchoke★★★/*Topinambour*: vegetable plant from which we eat the tubers. Green vegetable.

**Sunchoke chips/*Chips de topinambour*: very thinly cut sunchoke, fried and salted.

**Sunflower oil★★/*Huile de tournesol*: fatty substance made of sunflower seeds.

**Sunflower seed★★★/*Graine de tournesol*: sunflower seed eaten grilled.

**Sunflower seed milk★★★/*Lait de graines de tournesol*: plant milk from sunflower seeds. Lactose-free. *Note: do not consume if it's sweetened.*

**Surimi★★★/*Surimi*: mix of fish flesh flavored with crab.

**Sushi★★★/*Sushi*: small rice ball wrapped with raw fish cut in thin slices and wrapped in a seaweed leaf.

**Sushi sauce★★★/*Sauce sushi*: fermented soy sauce.

Swaledale cheese
- Sweetened and semi-skimmed powder goat milk

Swaledale cheese★: raw cow's milk cheese. Dairy product.
Note: do not consume more than approximately ½ oz of cheese three times per week... and never at dinner.

Sweat★★★/*Etuvée (à l')*: cf. "Steam".

Sweet and sour sauce/*Sauce aigre douce*: tomato sauce lightly sweetened.

Sweet chestnut cream/*Crème de marron*: sweet chestnut spread.

Sweet corn kernel★★★/*Maïs doux en grain*: cereal from which we eat the cooked kernel. Carbohydrate. Gluten-free.

Sweet potato★★★/*Patate douce*: edible tuber. Carbohydrate.

Sweet potatoes chips/*Chips de patates douces*: very thinly cut sweet potatoes, fried and salted.

Sweet potato flour★★★/*Farine de patate douce*: powder made of the extraction of starch from sweet potatoes. Carbohydrate. Gluten-free.

Sweet shortcrust pastry/*Pâte sablée*: pastry made of flour, sugar, butter and eggs.

Sweet wine/*Vin moelleux*: white wine which contains between 10 and 45 grams of sugar per liter.

Sweetened and semi-skimmed powder cow's milk/*Lait de vache demi-écrémé en poudre sucré*: dehydrated semi-skimmed cow's milk with added sugar.

Sweetened and semi-skimmed powder goat milk/*Lait de chèvre demi-écrémé en poudre sucré*: dehydrated semi-skimmed goat milk with added sugar.

**Sweetened and semi-skimmed powder sheep milk
- Sweetened skimmed sheep milk yogurt**

Sweetened and semi-skimmed powder sheep milk/*Lait de brebis demi-écrémé en poudre sucré*: dehydrated semi-skimmed sheep milk with added sugar.

Sweetened condensed milk/*Lait concentré sucré*: agri-food transformation of the milk from the industry packed in metal box or in tube and sweetened.

Sweetened shoyu★/*Shoyu sucré*: fermented and sweetened soy bean sauce.

Sweetened skimmed cow's milk yogurt★/*Yaourt au lait de vache maigre sucré*: cow's milk which has been partially or completely skimmed before being fermented thanks to lactic acid bacteria and sweetened. Dairy product.

Sweetened skimmed goat milk yogurt★/*Yaourt au lait de chèvre maigre sucré*: goat milk which has been partially or completely skimmed before being fermented thanks to lactic acid bacteria and sweetened. Dairy product.

Sweetened skimmed powder goat milk★/*Lait de chèvre écrémé en poudre sucré*: dehydrated skimmed goat milk with added sugar.

Sweetened skimmed powder cow's milk★/*Lait de vache écrémé en poudre sucré*: dehydrated skimmed cow's milk with added sugar.

Sweetened skimmed powder sheep milk★/*Lait de brebis écrémé en poudre sucré*: dehydrated skimmed sheep milk with added sugar.

Sweetened skimmed sheep milk yogurt★/*Yaourt au lait de brebis maigre sucré*: sheep milk which has been partially or completely skimmed before being fermented thanks to lactic acid bacteria and sweetened. Dairy product.

Sweetened whole cow's milk in powder - Swiss cheese

Sweetened whole cow's milk in powder/*Lait de vache entier en poudre sucré*: dehydrated whole cow's milk with added sugar.

Sweetened whole goat milk in powder/*Lait de chèvre entier en poudre sucré*: dehydrated whole goat milk with added sugar.

Sweetened whole goat milk yogurt/*Yaourt au lait de chèvre entier nature sucré*: whole goat milk fermented thanks to lactic acid bacteria before being sweetened. Dairy product.

Sweetened whole sheep milk in powder/*Lait de brebis entier en poudre sucré*: dehydrated whole sheep milk with added sugar.

Sweetened whole sheep milk yogurt/*Yaourt au lait de brebis entier nature sucré*: whole sheep milk fermented thanks to lactic acid bacteria before being sweetened. Dairy product.

Sweetened 0% fat fruit yogurt★★★/*Yaourt aux fruits à 0% de matière grasse édulcoré*: skimmed cow's milk, goat milk or sheep milk fermented thanks to lactic acid bacteria and in which fruits have been added. Dairy product.

Sweetened 0% fat yogurt★★★/*Yaourt à 0% de matière grasse édulcoré*: skimmed cow's milk, goat milk or sheep milk fermented thanks to lactic acid bacteria before being sweetened, usually with fructose. Dairy product.

Sweetener★★★/*Edulcorant*: substance suggesting the taste of sugar without containing sugar. Acaloric.

Swiss cheese★: pasteurised cow's milk cheese. Dairy product.
Note: do not consume more than approximately ½ oz of cheese three times per week... and never at dinner.

Swiss dried beef★★/*Viande des grisons*: dried meat served in very thin slice.

Swordfish★★★/*Espadon*: fatty fish we can find in hot waters.
Note: cook it without fat: en papillote, in water, grill, roast...

Syrup/*Sirop*: solution made of water and sugar.

T

Tabasco/Tabasco: cf. "Chili pepper purée".

Tabbouleh★★★/*Taboulé*: mix of wheat semolina, tomatoes, onions, bell peppers, raisins and mint leaves with olive oil. Carbohydrate.

Table salt★★/*Sel de table*: sodium chloride used to season dishes.

Taco★★/*Taco*: corn flour crepe stuffed with meat, cheese and hot sauce. Carbohydrate. Gluten-free.

Tagine★★/*Tagine*: dish made of pieces of meat or fish braised with green vegetables and various dried fruits.
Note: do not consume more than approximately 4 oz of red meat twice per week.

Tahini/*Tahini*: cf. "Sesame cream".

Tamari/*Tamari*: cf. "Soy sauce".

Tamarillo★★★/*Tamarillo*: small exotic fruit from the tamarillo.

Tamarind fruit in light syrup/*Tamarin au sirop léger*: poached tamarind fruit preserved in more or less sugary water. Exotic fruit.

Tamarind fruit in syrup/*Tamarin au sirop*: poached tamarind fruit preserved in very sugary water. Exotic fruit.

Tanacetum balsamita★★★/*Balsamite*: plant which leaves you can use as a condiment.

Tango/*Tango*: beverage made of half beer and half grenadine syrup.

Tapenade★/*Tapenade*: condiment made of crushed black olives, capers and anchovies with olive oil.

Tapioca★★★/*Tapioca*: cassava starch. Gluten-free.

Tapioca pearl★★★/*Perle du japon*: pearl made of cassava starch.

Tap water★★★/*Eau du robinet*: water commonly drunk and coming from the faucet.

Taramasalata★/*Tarama*: mix of salted fish eggs, olive oil, bread crumb and lemon juice.

Taro(1)★★★/*Colocase*: tropical plant which edible rhizome is rich in starch and assimilated to a carbohydrate.

Taro(2)★★★/*Taro*: tropical plant grown for its edible tuber. Green vegetable.

Tarragon★★★/*Estragon*: aromatic plant used as a condiment.

Tartare of fatty fish★★★/*Poisson gras tartare*: ground fatty fish eaten raw.

Tartare of lean fish★★★/*Poisson maigre tartare*: ground lean fish eaten raw.

Tartar sauce★/*Sauce tartare*: very seasoned mayonnaise with onions, capers and herbs.

Tartiflette/*Tartiflette*: dish made of melted reblochon, potatoes, lardons and onions.

Teal★★★/*Sarcelle*: wild duck. Game.
Note: cook it without fat: en papillote, in water, grill, roast...

Teff flake★★★/*Flocon de teff*: small portion of dehydrated teff. Carbohydrate.

Teff flour★★★/*Farine de teff*: powder made of not whole-grain teff seed milling. Gluten-free.

Teleme cheese★: pasteurised cow's milk cheese. Dairy product.
Note: do not consume more than approximately ½ oz of cheese three times per week... and never at dinner.

Tempeh★★★/*Tempeh*: food product made of fermented mung beans.

Tench★★★/*Tanche*: freshwater fish with white flesh.
Note: cook it without fat: en papillote, in water, grill, roast...

Tête-de-Maure cheese★/*Tête-de-Maure*: cow's milk cheese wrapped in red paraffin wax. Dairy product.
Note: do not consume more than approximately ½ oz of cheese three times per week... and never at dinner.

Theine-free (tea)★★★/*Déthéiné (thé)*: tea from which the theine has been removed.
Note: do not consume if it's sweetened.

Thyme★★★/*Thym*: plant used as a spice.

Tilsit cheese★/*Tilsit*: hard cow's milk cheese. Dairy product.
Note: do not consume more than approximately ½ oz of cheese three times per week... and never at dinner.

Tinned shoulder★★★/*Noix d'épaule*: canned pork shoulder.
Note: cook it without fat: en papillote, in water, grill, roast...

Tiramisu/*Tiramisu*: dessert made of alternating layers of whipped mascarpone with egg yolks and cookies soaked in coffee, sprinkled with cocoa in powder.

Toast(1)★★★/*Pain grillé*: fresh white bread cut in slices and industrially or "homemade" toasted. Carbohydrate.

Toast(2)★★★/*Toast*: slice of toasted bread.

Toasted brioche/*Toast brioché*: slice of toasted brioche.

To fry/*Frire*: to cook food in a boiling fatty substance.

Tofu★★★*Tofu*: poached or grilled soybean dough.

Tofu sausage★★★/*Saucisse de tofu*: sausage made of soybean and vegetable oil.
Note: cook it without fat.

Tomato★★★/*Tomate*: vegetable plant producing this fruit considered as a green vegetable: tomato. Green vegetable.

Tomato juice★★★/*Jus de tomate*: juice made of the pressing of tomatoes.

Tomato paste★★★/*Concentré de tomate*: tomato purée sold in cans or in cartons.

Tomme de Brach★/*Tomme de Brach*: cow's milk cheese with parsley in it. Dairy product.
Note: do not consume more than approximately ½ oz of cheese three times per week... and never at dinner.

Tomme de Romans★/*Tomme de Romans*: soft cow's milk cheese. Dairy product.
Note: do not consume more than approximately ½ oz of cheese three times per week... and never at dinner.

Tomme de Savoie★/*Tomme de Savoie*: pressed raw cow's milk cheese. Dairy product.
Note: do not consume more than approximately ½ oz of cheese three times per week... and never at dinner.

Topside★★/*Tende de tranche*: piece of beef to simmer. Red meat.
Note: do not consume more than approximately 4 oz of red meat twice per week. Note: cook it without fat except with olive oil.

Tortilla★★★/*Tortilla*: small crepe made of corn flour. Carbohydrate. Gluten-free.

Tortilla chips/*Tortilla chips*: swollen and light biscuit for the aperitif.

Tripe★★★/*Tripes*: dish made of the stomach and various animal entrails as well as animal feet prepared in various ways. Offal.

Triple cream cheese/*Fromage triple crème*: cheese containing more than 75% of fats. Dairy product.

Tripoux★★★/*Tripoux*: dish made of mutton tripe simmered in sauce. Offal.

Trotter★/*Pied de porc*: pork foot. Offal.

Trout - Turkey and cheese escalope

Trout★★★/**_Truite_**: fatty freshwater fish.
Note: cook it without fat: en papillote, in water, grill, roast...

Trout eggs★★/**_Œufs de truite_**: trout eggs preserved in brine.

True cardamom★★★/**_Cardamone_**: spice.

True fera★★★/**_Féra_**: freshwater fish with white flesh.
Note: cook it without fat: en papillote, in water, grill, roast...

Truffle★★★/**_Truffe_**: edible underground mushroom.

Tuberose parsley★★★/**_Persil à grosse racine_**: vegetable plant grown for its edible root. Green vegetable.

Tunerous-rooted chervil: cf. "Chaerophyllum b."

Tuna and mayonnaise/_Thon à la mayonnaise_: tuna in a can with mayonnaise sauce.

Tuna in Catalan sauce★★★/**_Thon à la catalane_**: tuna in a can with Catalan sauce.

Tuna in oil★/**_Thon à l'huile_**: tuna in a can with vegetable oil.

Tuna in tomato sauce★★★/**_Thon à la tomate_**: tuna in a can with concentrated tomato sauce.

Tuna rillettes★★/**_Rillettes de thon_**: cooked meat made of tuna cooked in vegetable oil.

Turkey★★★/**_Dinde_**: poultry with white flesh.
Note: cook it without fat: in water, grill, roast...

Turkey and cheese escalope★/**_Cordon bleu de dinde_**: turkey escalope wrapped around ham and cheese.
Note: cook it without fat.

Turkey chick (roast)★★★/*Dindonneau (rôti de)*: roast made of lean turkey slices. Poultry.

Turkey tournedos★★★/*Tournedos de dinde*: round slice of turkey poult roast.
Note: cook it without fat: grill, roast...

Turkish delight/*Loukoum*: very sugary Eastern confection made of a pasted flavored with almonds, pistachios, etc.

Turmeric★★★/*Curcuma*: spice.

Turnip★★★/*Navet*: vegetable plant from which we eat the edible root. Green vegetable.

Turnip seed★★★/*Graine de navet*: turnip seed eaten crushed or germinated.

$\mathcal{U}$

UHT sterilized milk★★★/*Lait stérilisé UHT*: milk which has been thermally treated at 240°F during 15 seconds before being rapidly cooled.
Note: do not drink whole milk.

Umbrina★★★/*Ombrine*: saltwater fish with white flesh.
Note: cook it without fat: en papillote, in water, grill, roast...

Unleavened bread★★★/*Pain azyme*: bread without leaven nor yeast. Carbohydrate.

Unsalted butter★★/*Beurre doux*: unsalted dietary fats made from the cream of cow's milk.
Note: consume it in moderation. Do not cook with it. The less fat, the better!

$\mathcal{V}$

Vacherin(1)★/*Vacherin(1)*: soft cow's milk cheese with washed rind. Dairy product.
Note: do not consume more than approximately ½ oz of cheese three times per week... and never at dinner.

Vacherin(2)★/*Vacherin(2)*: half hard cow's milk cheese. Dairy product.
Note: do not consume more than approximately ½ oz of cheese three times per week... and never at dinner.

Valençay cheese★/*Valençay*: raw goat milk cheese in the shape of a pyramid. Dairy product.
Note: do not consume more than approximately ½ oz of cheese three times per week... and never at dinner.

Vanilla★★★/*Vanille*: fruit from the vanilla planifolia used to flavor pastries.

Vanilla sugar/*Sucre vanillé*: sugar with vanilla extracts.

Varech★★★/*Kelp*: edible seaweed.

Veal and cheese escalope★/*Cordon bleu de veau*: veal escalope wrapped around ham and cheese.
Note: cook it without fat.

Veal breast★★/*Poitrine de veau*: inferior part of the veal's rib cage to boil or to simmer.
Note: cook it without fat.

Veal fillet★★★/*Quasi de veau*: piece from the veal leg.
Note: cook it without fat: en papillote, in water, grill, roast...

Veal gristle★★★/*Tendron de veau*: part of the veal composed of the cartilagees which prolong the ribs.
Note: cook it without fat: en papillote, in water, grill, roast...

Veal kidney★★★/*Rognon de veau*: kidney of the veal. Offal.
Note: cook it without fat: en papillote, grill, roast...

Veal knuckle★★★/*Jarret de veau*: part of the leg behind the veal's knee joint. Meat to boil.

Veal liver★★★/*Foie de veau*: offal.
Note: cook it without fat: en papillote, grill, roast...

Veal loin★★★/*Longe de veau*: veal meat corresponding to the upper part of the cervical and lumbar areas.
Note: cook it without fat: en papillote, in water, grill, roast...

Veal (meat)/*Veau (viande de...)*: all unprepared nor transformed meats, plain, ready to be cooked and cut from veal. See each piece separately.

Veal neck★★★/*Collet de veau*: piece of veal meat to boil.
Note: cook it without fat.

Veal quenelle★★★/*Quenelle de veau*: veal stuffing thickened with eggs and bread crumb before being shaped in sausage.

Veal rib★★★/*Côte de veau*: piece of veal meat to grill.
Note: cook it without fat.

Veal rump★★★/*Culotte de veau*: piece of veal to roast.
Note: cook it without fat.

Veal scallop - Vegetable steak

Veal scallop★★★/*Noix de veau*: piece of veal served roasted or as a scallop.
Note: cook it without fat: en papillote, in water, grill, roast...

Veal spare ribs★★★/*Carré de veau*: piece of veal meat to simmer.
Note: cook it without fat.

Veal stock★★★/*Fond de veau*: brown stock made of veal stock.

Veal sweetbread★★★/*Ris de veau*: veal thymus. Offal.
Note: cook it without fat.

Vegan★/*Végétalien(ne)*: person who does not eat any animal-based food.

Vegetable fondue★/*Fondue de légumes*: dish made of vegetables slowly cooked in a fatty substance.

Vegetable fry fat★★/*Graisse à frire végétale*: block of vegetable fat, especially coconut oil and palm kernel oil, used to fry food.

Vegetable gelatin/*Gélatine végétale*: cf. "Agar-agar".

Vegetable julienne★★★/*Julienne de légumes*: mix of green vegetable cut in thin sticks.

Vegetable pancake to pan-fry★★/*Galette végétale à poêler*: food under the form of a steak made of cereals: quinoa and/or wheat and/or rice, etc. without meat.
Note: cook it without fat.

Vegetable steak★★/*Steak végétal*: cereal steak made of wheat and/or quinoa and/or soybean, etc. Meatless.
Note: cook it without fat.

Vegetable terrine★/*Pain de légumes*: dish made of potatoes, green vegetables, butter and eggs served cold with a mayonnaise.

Vegetarian oyster sauce★★★/*Sauce d'huître végétarienne*: sauce made of shiitakes (black mushrooms) stock reduction.

Vegetarian★★/*Végétarien(ne)*: person who does not eat meat nor fish nor any transformed dish or product containing meat or fish.

Venison (meat)★★/*Chevreuil (viande de...)*: red meat and game.
Note: do not consume more than approximately 4 oz of red meat twice per week. Cook it without fat: en papillote, in water, grill, roast...

Venison★★/*Venaison*: edible flesh from big games (wild boar, deer, hind, etc.)
Note: cook it without fat: en papillote, in water, grill, roast... Do not consume more than approximately 4 oz of red meat twice per week.

Ventreche★/*Ventrèche*: lean lard.
Note: cook it without fat: grill, roast...

Verbena★★★/*Verveine*: plant used as a condiment and eaten in infusions.
Note: do not consume if it's sweetened.

Vermicelli(1)/*Vermicelle*: sweetened chestnut pasta in the shape of a thin filament.

Vermicelli(2)/*Vermicelle de "..."*: cf. ""..." pasta".

Very rare★/*Bleu*: cooking method during which the red meat remains bloody.
Note: do not consume more than approximately ½ oz of cheese three times per week... and never at dinner.

Vienna bread/*Pain viennois*: bread which batter contains sugar, milk, fats and eggs.

Viennoiserie/*Viennoiserie*: bakery product made of a fermented dough with milk, sugar, fats and eggs.

Vieux-Lille cheese★/*Vieux-Lille*: very fermented raw cow's milk cheese. Dairy product.
Note: do not consume more than approximately ½ oz of cheese three times per week... and never at dinner.

Vila-vila★★★/*Morelle de Balbis*: plant from which we eat the small fruits.

Vinaigrette sauce★★/*Sauce vinaigrette*: sauce made of vegetable oil and vinegar.

Vinegar★★★/*Vinaigre*: aqueous sour solution made of a fermented alcoholic beverage.

Vodka/*Vodka*: eau de vie made of wheat and rye seeds.

W

Waffle★★/*Gaufre*: light honeycombed pastry.
Note: do not consume if it's sweetened.

Wakame★★★/*Wakamé*: edible seaweed.

Wakame pasta★★★/*Pâte alimentaire de wakamé*: mix to be cooked made of wakame (edible seaweed). Green vegetable.

Walleye★★★/*Doré*: freshwater fish very similar to zander.
Note: cook it without fat: en papillote, in water, grill, roast...

Walnut★★/*Noix*: nut from the walnut tree.

Walnut oil★★/*Huile de noix*: fatty substance made of walnut.

Warp★★★/*Warp*: sieved wheat pancake. Carbohydrate.

Wasabi★★★/*Wasabi*: Japanese mustard.

Watercress★★★/*Cresson*: plant grown for its edible leaves. Green vegetable.

Watercress seed★★★/*Graine de cresson*: watercress seed eaten crushed or germinated.

Waterloo cheese★: raw cow's milk cheese. Dairy product.
Note: do not consume more than approximately ½ oz of cheese three times per week... and never at dinner.

Watermelon in light syrup/*Pastèque au sirop léger*: poached watermelon preserved in more or less sugary water.

Watermelon in syrup/*Pastèque au sirop*: poached watermelon preserved in very sugary water.

Watermelon juice★/*Jus de pastèque*: juice made of the pressing of watermelons.

Wax bean★★★/*Haricot beurre*: yellow bean eaten young. Green vegetable.

Wedge sole★★★/*Céteau*: small sole, flat saltwater fish with white flesh.
Note: cook it without fat: en papillote, in water, grill, roast...

Weever★★★/*Vive*: saltwater fish with white flesh.
Note: cook it without fat: en papillote, in water, grill, roast...

Wheat bran★★★/*Son de blé*: residue of wheat milling.

Wheat bread industrially toasted★★/*Pain de froment grillé industriel*: white bread slice industrially toasted.

Wheat crispbread★★/*Biscotte de froment*: slice of sandwich bread industrially toasted in the oven. Carbohydrate.

Wheat germ oil★★/*Huile de germe de blé*: fatty substance made of wheat germ.

Wheat gluten★★★/*Seitan*: food product made of wheat proteins.

Wheat pasta★★★/*Pâte alimentaire de blé*: mix to be cooked made of refined hard wheat semolina. Carbohydrate.

Wheat tunnbröd★★/*Pain suédois au froment*: small dry bread made of soft wheat flour. Carbohydrate.

Wheat(1)★★★/*Blé(1)*: herbaceous plant from which the grain is extracted to make wheat flour used to make bread and pasta, etc. Carbohydrate.

Wheat(2)★★★/*Blé(2)*: pre-cooked whole wheat. Carbohydrate.

Wheat★★/*Froment*: soft wheat. Carbohydrate.

Wheatgerm★★★/*Germe de blé*: wheat germ sold loose.

Whelk★★/*Bulot* : sea shellfish.
Note: cook it without fat: in water, grill ...

Whipped cream/*Crème Chantilly*: whipped crème fraîche with sugar.

Whipped egg whites★★★/***Œuf monté en neige***: egg white whipped until firm and foamy.

Whipping cream★★/***Crème fleurette***: cream with 10 to 12% of fats. Made of sterilized UHT milk. Dairy product.

Whiskey/*Whisky*: grain eau de vie.

White barley flour★★★/***Farine d'orge blanche***: powder made of not whole-grain barley milling. Carbohydrate.

White bread★★/***Pain blanc***: bread made of white or sieved flour. Carbohydrate.

White bread crumb★/***Mie de pain blanc***: bread made of white flour without its crust. Carbohydrate.

White buckwheat flour★★★/***Farine de sarrasin blanche***: powder made of not whole-grain buckwheat milling. Carbohydrate.

White chocolate/*Chocolat blanc*: confection made of fats, dairy products and sugar. Does not contain cocoa powder.

White einkorn wheat flour★★★/***Farine de petit épeautre blanche***: powder made of not whole-grain einkorn wheat milling. Carbohydrate.

White flour★★★/***Farine blanche***: flour made of grains without their peel. Only starch is kept. It is thus very poor in fiber. T45 to T80 flour in Europe. Carbohydrate.

White fonio★★★/***Fonio***: very thin grain. Carbohydrate. Gluten-free.

White fonio flake★★★/***Flocon de fonio***: small portion of dehydrated white fonio. Carbohydrate. Gluten-free.

White meat - White wheat flour

White meat★★★/*Viande blanche*: poultry, veal, pork, rabbit meat.
Note: cook it without fat: en papillote, in water, grill, roast...

White millet flour★★★/*Farine de millet blanche*: powder made of not whole-grain millet milling. Carbohydrate.

White oats flour★★★/*Farine d'avoine blanche*: powder made of not wholewheat oats milling. Carbohydrate.

White rice★★★/*Riz blanc*: rice without peel and without bran. Carbohydrate. Gluten-free.

White rye flour★★★/*Farine de seigle blanche*: powder made of not whole-grain rye milling. Carbohydrate.

White sauce★★/*Sauce blanche*: white roux made of fat and flour.

White sausage★★★/*Boudin blanc*: cooked meat made of lean meat stuffing, milk, eggs, cream, bread crumbs or flour and spices.
Note: cook it without fat: en papillote, in water, grill...

White spelt flour★★★/*Farine d'épeautre blanche*: powder made of not whole-grain spelt milling. Carbohydrate.

White sugar/*Sucre blanc*: very sugary substance extracted from sugar cane and/or sugar beet. Fast-acting sugar.

White tea★★★/*Thé blanc*: infusion of white tea leaves.
Note: do not consume if it's sweetened.

White wheat flour★★★/*Farine de blé blanche*: powder made of not wholewheat milling. Carbohydrate.

White wine★/*Vin blanc*: wine made thanks of the grape must alcoholic fermentation.
Note: do not drink alcoholic beverage, however no problem if it's cooked.

Whiting★★★/*Merlan*: saltwater fish with white flesh.
Note: cook it without fat: en papillote, in water, grill, roast...

Whole cow's milk/*Lait de vache entier*: cow's milk which has not been skimmed.

Whole goat milk/*Lait de chèvre entier*: goat milk which has not been skimmed.

Whole sheep milk/*Lait de brebis entier*: sheep milk which has not been skimmed.

Whole tomato preserved peeled★★★/*Tomate entière pelée en conserve*: peeled tomato preserved in brine.

Whole-grain almond purée★★/*Purée d'amande complète*: mashed whole-grain almonds to spread.

Whole-grain and gluten-free bagel★★★/*Bagel complet sans gluten*: small whole-grain bread shaped into a ring with very firm gluten-free crumb. Carbohydrate.

Whole-grain bagel★★★/*Bagel complet*: small whole-grain bread shaped into a ring with very firm crumb. Carbohydrate.

Whole-grain barley flake★★★/*Flocon d'orge complète*: small portion of dehydrated whole-grain barley. Carbohydrate.

Whole-grain barley flour★★★/*Farine d'orge complète*: powder made of whole-grain barley milling. Carbohydrate.

**Whole-grain breakfast cookie
- Whole-grain corn flour**

Whole-grain breakfast cookie★/*Biscuit pour petit-déjeuner riche en céréales complètes*: cookie rich in whole grains and adapted to breakfast. Carbohydrate.

Whole-grain buckwheat cornflakes★★/*Corn flakes de sarrasin complet*: grilled flakes made of whole-grain buckwheat flakes. Carbohydrate. Gluten-free.
Note: do not consume if it's sweetened.

Whole-grain buckwheat flake★★★/*Flocon de sarrasin complet*: small portion of dehydrated whole-grain buckwheat. Carbohydrate.

Whole-grain buckwheat flour★★★/*Farine de sarrasin complète*: powder made of whole-grain buckwheat milling. Carbohydrate.

Whole-grain buckwheat pancake★★★/*Galette complète*: flat, thin and round dish made of whole-grain buckwheat flour, eggs and milk cooked in a frying pan. Carbohydrate. Gluten-free.

Whole-grain cannellonis★★★/*Cannelloni complet*: whole-grain pasta rolled in the shape of a cylinder and stuffed with stuffing. Carbohydrate.

Whole-grain cashew purée★★/*Purée de noix de cajou complète*: mashed whole-grain cashew to spread.

Whole-grain corn cornflakes★★/*Corn flakes de maïs complet*: grilled flakes made of whole-grain corn corn flakes. Carbohydrate. Gluten-free.
Note: do not consume if it's sweetened.

Whole-grain corn flake★★★/*Flocon de maïs complet*: small portion of dehydrated whole-grain corn. Carbohydrate. Gluten-free.

Whole-grain corn flour★★★/*Farine de maïs complète*: powder made of whole-grain corn milling. Carbohydrate. Gluten-free.

Whole-grain crispbread★★/*Biscotte complète*: slice of whole-grain sandwich bread industrially toasted in the oven. Carbohydrate.

Whole-grain einkorn wheat flake★★★/*Flocon de petit-épeautre complet*: small portion of dehydrated whole-grain einkorn wheat. Carbohydrate.

Whole-grain einkorn wheat flour★★★/*Farine de petit épeautre complet*: powder made of whole-grain einkorn wheat milling. Carbohydrate.

Whole-grain fajita★★★/*Fajita complète*: whole-grain corn tortilla. Carbohydrate. Gluten-free.

Whole-grain fonio flake★★★/*Flocon de fonio complète*: small portion of dehydrated whole-grain fonio. Carbohydrate. Gluten-free.

Whole-grain frik★★★/*Frik complet*: crushed not fully grown whole-grain wheat. Carbohydrate.

Whole-grain gluten-free crispbread★★/*Biscotte complète sans gluten*: slice of whole-grain gluten-free sandwich bread industrially toasted in the oven. Carbohydrate.

Whole-grain gluten-free kringle★★★/*Craquelin complet sans gluten*: small whole-grain crispy cookie made of an unleavened and gluten-free batter.

Whole-grain gnocchi★★★/*Gnocchi complet*: ball made of wholewheat semolina and potatoes. Carbohydrate.

Whole-grain grissino★★★/*Gressin complet*: small whole-grain bread made with an egg batter. Carbohydrate.

Whole-grain hazelnut purée★★/*Purée de noisette complète*: mashed whole-grain hazelnuts to spread.

**Whole-grain khorasan wheat flake
- Whole-grain fonio flour**

Whole-grain khorasan wheat flake★★★/***Flocon de kamut complet***: small portion of dehydrated whole-grain khorasan wheat. Carbohydrate.

Whole-grain khorasan wheat flour★★★/***Farine de kamut complète***: powder made of whole-grain khorasan wheat milling. Carbohydrate.

Whole-grain kringle★★/***Craquelin complet***: small whole-grain crispy cookie made of an unleavened batter.

Whole-grain millet flake★★★/***Flocon de millet complet***: small portion of dehydrated whole-grain millet. Carbohydrate. Gluten-free.

Whole-grain millet flour★★★/***Farine de millet complète***: powder made of whole-grain millet milling. Carbohydrate.

Whole-grain millet slice of bread★★/***Tartine craquante millet complète***: flat and light slice of bread made of whole-grain millet flour. Carbohydrate. Gluten-free.

Whole-grain milliasse★★★/***Milliasse complète***: mash made of whole-grain corn flour before being cooled and grilled. Carbohydrate. Gluten-free.

Whole-grain muffin★★★/***Muffin complet***: small plain whole-grain bread with leaven. Carbohydrate.

Wholegrain mustard★★★/***Moutarde à l'ancienne***: mustard with its seeds.

Whole-grain oats flour★★★/***Farine d'avoine complète***: powder made of whole-grain oats milling. Carbohydrate.

Whole-grain fonio flour★★★/***Farine de fonio complète***: powder made of whole-grain folio milling. Carbohydrate. Gluten-free.

Whole-grain peanut purée★★/*Purée d'arachide complète*: mashed whole-grain peanuts to spread.

Whole-grain pistachio purée★★/*Purée de pistache complète*: mashed whole-grain pistachios to spread.

Whole-grain polenta★★★/*Polenta complète*: whole-grain corn mush. Gluten-free.

Whole-grain quinoa flour★★★/*Farine de quinoa complète*: flour made of whole-grain quinoa seed milling. Gluten-free.

Whole-grain rice★★★/*Riz complet*: rice eaten intact without its peel. Carbohydrate. Gluten-free.

Whole-grain rice bulgur★★★/*Boulgour de riz complet*: crushed whole-grain rice steamed or cooked in water. Carbohydrate. Gluten-free.

Whole-grain rice cornflakes★★/*Corn flakes de riz complet*: grilled flakes made of whole-grain rice flakes. Carbohydrate. Gluten-free.
Note: do not consume if it's sweetened.

Whole-grain rice cream★★★/*Crème de riz complet*: more or less liquid cream made of whole-grain rice milk, substitute to crème fraîche.

Whole-grain rice flake★★★/*Flocon de riz complet*: small portion of dehydrated whole-grain rice. Carbohydrate. Gluten-free.

Whole-grain rice flour★★★/*Farine de riz complet*: powder made of whole-grain rice milling. Carbohydrate. Gluten-free.

Whole-grain rye flake★★★/*Flocon de seigle complet*: small portion of dehydrated whole-grain rye. Carbohydrate.

Whole-grain rye flour★★★/*Farine de seigle complète*: powder made of whole-grain rye milling. Carbohydrate.

Whole-grain salt-free & gluten-free crispbread★★/*Biscotte complète sans sel & sans gluten*: slice of whole-grain gluten-free and salt-free sandwich bread industrially toasted in the oven. Carbohydrate.

Whole-grain soybean flake★★★/*Flocon de soja complet*: small portion of dehydrated whole-grain soybean. Carbohydrate.

Whole-grain soybean flour★★★/*Farine de soja complète*: flour made of whole-grain soybean milling. Gluten-free.

Whole-grain spelt cornflakes★★/*Corn flakes d'épeautre complet*: grilled flakes made of whole-grain spelt flakes. Carbohydrate.
Note: do not consume if it's sweetened.

Whole-grain spelt flake★★★/*Flocon d'épeautre complet*: small portion of dehydrated whole-grain spelt. Carbohydrate.

Whole-grain spelt flour★★★/*Farine d'épeautre complète*: powder from whole-grain spelt milling. Carbohydrate.

Whole-grain teff flake★★★/*Flocon de teff complet*: small portion of dehydrated whole-grain teff. Carbohydrate.

Whole-grain teff flour★★★/*Farine de teff complète*: flour made of whole-grain teff seed milling. Gluten-free.

Whole-grain tortilla★★★/*Tortilla complète*: small crepe made of whole wheat corn flour. Carbohydrate. Gluten-free.

Whole-grain amaranth flour★★★/*Farine d'amarante complète*: flour made of whole-grain amaranth milling. Gluten-free.

Wholewheat bread★★★/*Pain complet*: bread made of wholewheat or semi wholewheat flour. Carbohydrate.

Wholewheat bread crumb★★★/*Mie de pain complet*: bread made of wholewheat flour without its crust. Carbohydrate.

Wholewheat breadcrumbs★★★/*Chapelure complète*: wholewheat bread toasted in the oven before being crushed into crumbs. Carbohydrate.

Wholewheat bread industrially toasted★★★/*Pain complet grillé industriel*: wholewheat bread slice industrially toasted.

Wholewheat bulgur★★★/*Boulgour complet*: crushed whole wheat steamed or cooked in water. Carbohydrate.

Wholewheat bun★★★/*Bun complet*: small round and puffy wholewheat bread. Carbohydrate.

Wholewheat crepe★★★/*Crêpe complète*: thin layer of cooked batter made of eggs, milk and wholewheat flour. Carbohydrate.
Note: do not consume if it's sweetened.

Wholewheat crouton★★★/*Croûton complet*: small piece of fried wholewheat bread. Carbohydrate.

Wholemeal flour★★★/*Farine complète:* flour made of whole-grains or almost whole grains. It is thus rich in fiber.

Wholewheat flour(1)★★★/*Farine complète:* flour made of whole-grains or almost whole grains. It is thus rich in fiber.

Wholewheat flour - Wholewheat wrap

Wholewheat flour(2)★★★/*Farine de blé complète*:
powder made of wholewheat milling. Carbohydrate.

Wholewheat gluten-free bun★★★/*Bun complet sans gluten*: small round and puffy gluten-free wholewheat bread. Carbohydrate.

Wholewheat lasagna★★★/*Lasagne complète*: pasta made of wholewheat flour in the shape of large flat patches. Carbohydrate.

Wholewheat macaroni★★★/*Macaroni complet*: wholewheat semolina pasta in the shape of a tube. Carbohydrate.

Wholewheat pancakes★★★/*Pancakes complet*: small thick crepes made of wholewheat flour. Carbohydrate. *Note: do not consume if it's sweetened.*

Wholewheat peanut flour★★/*Farine d'arachide complète*: flour made of wholewheat peanut milling. Gluten-free.

Wholewheat pitta★★★/*Pita complet*: unleavened wholewheat bread. Carbohydrate.

Wholewheat toast(1)★★★/*Pain grillé complet*: fresh wholewheat bread cut in slices and industrially or "homemade" toasted. Carbohydrate.

Wholewheat toast(2)★★★/*Toast complet*: slice of wholewheat toasted bread.

Wholewheat tunnbröd★★★/*Pain suédois complet*: small dry bread made of wholewheat flour. Carbohydrate.

Wholewheat wrap★★★/*Warp complet*: wholewheat pancake. Carbohydrate.

Wild boar (meat)★★★/*Sanglier (viande de...)*: untransformed and unprepared plain meats, ready to be cooked and coming from the wild boar. Game.
Note: cook it without fat: en papillote, in water, grill, roast...

Wild rabbit★★★/*Lapin sauvage*: herbivore mammal.
Note: cook it without fat: en papillote, in water, grill, roast...

Wild rice/*Riz sauvage*: cf. "Whole-grain rice".

Williamine★/*Williamine*: pear eau de vie.
Note: do not drink alcoholic beverage, however no problem if it's cooked.

Wine beef fondue★★/*Fondue bourguignonne au vin*: dish made of small dices of beef dipped in boiling wine. Red meat.
Note: do not consume more than approximately 4 oz of red meat twice per week.

Winkle★★★/*Bigorneau*: edible mollusk.
Note: cook it without fat: grill, in water....

Winter purslane: cf. "Claytonia perfoliata".

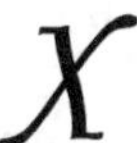

Xylitol★★★/*Xylitol*: alcohol-sugar used as a sweetener.

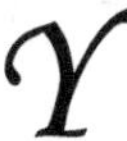

Yacón★★★/*Poire de terre*: vegetable plant from which we eat the tubers. Carbohydrate. Gluten-free.

Yakitori sauce★/*Sauce yakitori*: fermented and sweetened soy sauce.

Yam★★★/*Igname*: vegetable plant grown for its rhizome. Green vegetable.

Yam flake★★★/*Flocon d'igname*: small portion of dehydrated yam. Carbohydrate.

Yam flour★★★/*Farine d'igname*: powder made of yam milling. Carbohydrate. Gluten-free.

Yannoh★★★/*Yannoh*: beverage made of rye, curly endive, acorn and barley.
Note: do not consume if it's sweetened.

Yogurt rich in phytosterol★★★/*Yaourt riche en phytostérols*: cow's milk, goat milk or sheep milk fermented thanks to lactic acid bacteria before being enriched with phytosterol. Dairy product.
Note: do not consume if it's sweetened.

Yogurt with cereals★★★/*Yaourt aux céréales*: sweetened yogurt with various cereals in powder.
Note: do not consume if it's sweetened.

Yogurt with muesli : cf. "Yogurt with cereals".

York ham★★★/*Jambon d'York*: pork ham cooked with its bone. Cooked meat.
Note: cook it without fat: en papillote, in water, grill, roast...

Young rooster★★★/*Coquelet*: young hen or young chicken. Poultry.
Note: cook it without fat: en papillote, in water, grill, roast...

Z

Zander★★★/*Sandre*: freshwater fish with white flesh. *Note: cook it without fat: en papillote, in water, grill, roast...*

0% fat cow's milk cottage cheese★★★/*Faisselle au lait de vache à 0% de matière grasse*: fresh cheese made of skimmed cow's milk. Dairy product.

0% fat cow's milk fromage blanc★★★/*Fromage blanc de vache à 0% de matière grasse*: fresh cheese made of skimmed cow's milk, a bit drained and not aged. Dairy product.

0% fat goat milk cottage cheese★★★/*Faisselle au lait de chèvre à 0% de matière grasse*: fresh cheese made of skimmed goat milk. Dairy product.

0% fat goat milk fromage blanc★★★/*Fromage blanc de chèvre à 0% de matière grasse*: fresh cheese made of skimmed goat milk, a bit drained and not aged. Dairy product.

0% fat sheep milk cottage cheese★★★/*Faisselle au lait de brebis à 0% de matière grasse*: fresh cheese made of skimmed sheep milk. Dairy product.

0% fat sheep milk fromage blanc★★★/*Fromage blanc de brebis à 0% de matière grasse*: fresh cheese made of skimmed sheep milk, a bit drained and not aged. Dairy product.

0% fat yogurt with sugar★/*Yaourt à 0% de matière grasse sucré*: skimmed cow's milk, goat milk or sheep milk fermented thanks to lactic acid bacteria and in which sugar is added. Dairy product.

0% sugar syrup★★★/*Sirop 0% de sucre*: syrup made of sweetener, usually stevia extracts.

Zerumbet★★★/*Zérumbet*: aromatic rhizome close to ginger. Green vegetable.

Zest★★★/*Zeste*: external peel of citrus fruits.

Zucchini★★★/*Courgette*: kind of squash with round and long fruit. Green vegetable.

All books by Ménard Cédric

Culinary dictionary for osteoporosis.
Culinary dictionary forcolonic diverticula.
Culinary dictionary for constipation.
Culinary dictionary for a food without gluten.
Culinary dictionary for anemia.
Culinary dictionary forangina pectoris.
Culinary dictionary for calcium oxalate kidney stones.
Culinary dictionary for corticosteroid therapy.
Culinary dictionary for diarrhea.
Culinary dictionary for diet without lactose.
Culinary dictionary for gastritis.
Culinary dictionary for gastroesophageal reflux disease.
Culinary dictionary for gout.
Culinary dictionary for hypercholesterolemia.
Culinary dictionary for heart failure.
Culinary dictionary for hemochromatosis.
Culinary dictionary for hiatal hernia.
Culinary dictionary for hypothyroidism.
Culinary dictionary for indigestion (or dyspepsia).
Culinary dictionary for lose weight.
Culinary dictionary for low sodium diet.
Culinary dictionary for myocardial infarction.
Culinary dictionary for breastfeeding.
Culinary dictionary of nutritional valueof food.
Culinary dictionary for diabetes mellitus.
Culinary dictionary for healthy pregnant woman.
Culinary dictionary for ulcerative colitis.
Culinary dictionary for uric acid kidney stones.
Culinary dictionary for theCrohn's disease.
Culinary dictionary for pancreatitis.
Culinary dictionary for cystic fibrosis.
Recipes and menusfor ulcerative colitis.
Recipes and menus for the Crohn's disease.